19.50

D0856057

# STATE MENTAL HOSPITALS

What Happens When They Close

# Current Topics in Mental Health

Series Editors:   Paul I. Ahmed
*Southeastern University*

and

Stanley C. Plog
*Plog Research, Inc.*

---

STATE MENTAL HOSPITALS: What Happens When They Close
Edited by Paul I. Ahmed and Stanley C. Plog

COPING WITH PHYSICAL ILLNESS
Edited by Rudolf H. Moos

*In preparation:*

THE PRINCIPLES AND TECHNIQUES OF MENTAL HEALTH CONSULTATION
Edited by Stanley C. Plog and Paul I. Ahmed

# STATE MENTAL HOSPITALS

## What Happens When They Close

Edited by

### Paul I. Ahmed
*Southeastern University*
*Washington, D.C.*

and

### Stanley C. Plog
*Plog Research, Inc.*
*Reseda (Los Angeles), California*

PLENUM MEDICAL BOOK COMPANY
New York and London

Library of Congress Cataloging in Publication Data

Main entry under title:

State mental hospitals, what happens when they close.

(Current topics in mental health)
Includes bibliographical references and index.
1. Psychiatric hospitals. 2. Community mental health services. I. Ahmed, Paul I. II.
Plog, Stanley C. [DNLM: 1. Hospitals, Psychiatric—Supply and distribution—United
States. 2. Community mental health services—United States. WM27 AA1 S78]
RC439.S78                   362.1 1'0973                        76-21706
ISBN 0-306-30897-5

© 1976 Plenum Publishing Corporation
227 West 17th Street, New York, N.Y. 10011

Plenum Medical Book Company is an imprint of Plenum Publishing Corporation

Printed in the United States of America

To

the memory of the

late Dr. Zakir Husain

former president of India

a wise teacher, a warm friend,

an inspiring leader,

and a great human being

# Preface

The 1970s constitute the decade of decisions about state mental hospitals! These large, monolithic, and seemingly impervious institutions are being phased out in some states and their basic purpose for existence is being seriously questioned in almost all others. Since 1970, hospitals have closed in California, Illinois, Kentucky, Massachusetts, Minnesota, New York, Oklahoma, Washington, and Wisconsin. Similar closings have occurred in several provinces of Canada, in Great Britain, and in some European countries.

The purpose of the book is to examine the multiple issues growing out of the hospital closings:

Why are the state hospitals being closed?

What is the impact of closings on patients, hospital staff, and the communities where the hospitals are located?

What has been the impact on the communities receiving these patients?

What are the trends for the future, in terms of numbers of closings and types of hospitals which will remain?

Is there a role for the state hospital in the care of the mentally ill or is it an obsolete institution?

The impetus for the closings is diverse. The discovery and widespread use of the tranquilizing drugs in the early 1950s allowed more patients to be returned to the community—under medication. The Community Mental Health Centers Act of 1963 provided for the development of more than 500 community mental health centers (CMHCs) across the nation with the basic responsibility of serving troubled people within the communities where they live, rather than passing them on to the state hospital system. And, the general growth of more recent humanitarian and consumer-based social movements has led to greater concern about the rights of mental patients and how these rights are often violated through involuntary hospitalization.

But there is considerable controversy surrounding the issue. Is community care a better form of treatment than hospitalization? How adequate are the community facilities and who will supervise them? Does the public want mental hospital patients roaming around the streets? What will happen to persons who require custodial or 24-hour care—severely mentally retarded, schizophrenics, long-term alcoholics, for example? Have the legal rights of patients been protected as they have been moved out of state hospitals?

These and other questions need answers. The editors hope that the present work will provide these answers for many of the questions raised and stimulate a further exchange of ideas and information in the field. It is hoped, too, that the issues raised here will lead to further investigation into those areas where sufficient data are lacking. The timeliness of the present book derives from the fact that major decisions are now being made and are affecting the lives of mental patients, their families, and taxpayers, but without the benefit of information necessary for effective planning.

The book presents a balanced view. Our purpose is not to support the existence or nonexistence of state hospitals or the adequacy or inadequacy of community care facilities. Rather, our aim is to present all sides of the question. There are no clear-cut answers or solutions. What is needed is information to assist others in making up their own minds about these critical issues.

The collection of authors is outstanding, representing well-known specialists who have written previously about mental hospitals, pragmatists who have supervised hospital closings, researchers who have investigated the impact of these closings, and community specialists. All authors were requested to present their views as forcefully as possible to support their arguments vigorously, and to offer readers a clear understanding of the major issues in the field. As a result, it is hoped, the book will be a lively and readable overview of the problems involved in state hospital closings.

Special thanks are due to the authors, who devoted considerable energy and time to writing the papers included in this book. Their cooperation in revising their papers, in meeting deadlines when requested, and in producing scholarly work is deeply appreciated. Thanks are also due to Nancy Ahmed, who did support work and typing for the publication of the book, and to Natalie Gawdiak for her assistance in preparing the manuscript. Special thanks are due to Diane Drobnis, senior editor of Plenum Publishing Corporation, who always gave a helping hand and advice on all matters pertaining to the publication of this work.

PAUL I. AHMED
STANLEY E. PLOG
*Editors*

# Contributors

Paul I. Ahmed, M.A., L.L.B.   *Professor, Southeastern University, Washington, D. C.*

Uri Aviram, Ph.D.   *Tel Aviv University, Tel Aviv, Israel.*

Leo Barrington, Ph.D.   *Assistant Professor, Regis College, Weston, Massachusetts, and Social Scientist, World Health Organization, Ghana, Africa.*

John H. Cumming, M.D.   *Mental Health Branch, Department of Health Services and Health Insurance, Victoria, British Columbia.*

Paul R. Dingman, Ph.D.   *Director, University Counselling Center, Colgate University, Hamilton, New York.*

Elizabeth Glazier, MPH   *Staff Epidemiologist, Department of Psychiatry, Veterans Administration Hospital, Sepulveda, California, and Assistant Professor, California State University, Northridge, California.*

Milton Greenblatt, M.D.   *Professor of Psychiatry, University of California, Los Angeles, California, and Chief of Psychiatry, Veterans Administration Hospital, Sepulveda, California.*

Frederic Grunberg, M.D., D.P.M.   *Associate Professor of Psychiatry, Albany Medical College, Union University, Jackson, Tennessee, and Chief, Inpatient Services, Albany Medical Center, Albany, New York.*

Hugh G. Lafave, M.D., C.M.   *Eleanor Roosevelt Developmental Services, Schenectady, New York.*

Elizabeth W. Markson, Ph.D.   *Division of Research and Evaluation, Massachusetts Department of Mental Health, Boston, Massachusetts.*

Roberta A. Marlowe, Ph.D.   *Department of Health of the State of California, Sacramento, California.*

Werner M. Mendel, M.D.   *Professor of Psychiatry, University of Southern California School of Medicine, Los Angeles, California.*

Stanley C. Plog, Ph.D.   *Plog Inc., Encino, California.*

**Stephen Rachlin, M.D.**   *Deputy Director, Meyer-Manhattan Psychiatric Center, Ward's Island, New York, and Assistant Clinical Professor of Psychiatry, Columbia University College of Physicians and Surgeons, New York.*

**Jonas Robitscher, J.D., M.D.**   *Henry R. Luce Professor of Law and the Behavioral Sciences, Emory University, Atlanta, Georgia.*

**Steven P. Segal, Ph.D.**   *School of Social Welfare, University of California, Berkeley, California.*

**Samuel Weiner, M.A.**   *Economist, Stanford Research Institute, Menlo Park, California.*

**Richard W. Woodhouse, Ph.D.**   *Eleanor Roosevelt Developmental Services, Schenectady, New York.*

# Contents

# I

# Perspectives in the Closing of Mental Hospitals

# 1

# Introduction and an Overview of the Closing Scene

PAUL I. AHMED AND STANLEY C. PLOG

This is a book about a movement—a movement begun by Dorothea Dix that started as the hope of the future for the mentally disturbed, and is now ending with hopes shattered and expectations unmet, under the aegis of judicial scrutiny, and with public outcry. The mental hospital, as an institution, is under fire, not for what it has done for the mentally disturbed and ill but for what it has not done. Legislators, judges, community workers, mayors, and even the Supreme Court are involved in the fight. Although the outcome of what has been a protracted struggle is in doubt, the beginning of the end is in sight. The mental hospital, as constituted in the early 20th century, is dead. A new definition of mental hospital is emerging which will continue to be reshaped on the basis of judicial adjudication and public scrutiny.

There are many indications of what is to come. After a period of growth, state institutions for the mentally ill and mentally disturbed and retarded are being curtailed, converted to new uses and, in some cases, closed. Inpatient census figures are on the decline and the cost per patient served is on the rise. Both Congress and the federal bureaucracy by their actions and appropriations have indicated that they look at these changes favorably. The judicial system has also been attacking

PAUL I. AHMED • Professor, Southeastern University, Washington, D.C. 20024.
STANLEY C. PLOG • Plog Inc., Encino, California 91316.

these institutions, thus helping the direction of the movement of closing.

The movement toward hospital closings started in the early 1960s
in California. Because of the age of the buildings at Modesto State
Hospital (built as barracks during World War II), considerable discussion developed over the possibility of closing the institution. This move
was given further impetus with the passage of the Lanterman–Petris–
Short Act, which limited the use of involuntary commitment. And,
under the cost-cutting directives of a new fiscally conservative governor, Ronald Reagan, the California Department of Mental Hygiene
made a concerted effort to step up hospital discharges and to support
the expansion of Comprehensive Community Mental Health Care
(CCMHC) services.

In 1969 the planned closing of Modesto State Hospital was
announced and, over a period of one year, all patients were transferred
to other hospitals. The senior editor of this book completed a study of
Modesto which indicated that very few staff members lost their jobs
and, in general, the patient relocation process went well. On the community side of the issue, no decline in business was measured, bank
deposits remained high, real estate sales were up, and the real impact of
the loss of this major industry in a small town was felt by those who had
to relocate. The state offered the majority of employees jobs at Stockton
Hospital, which were accepted by most, thereby enabling them to
maintain their residences in Modesto.

In 1970 California announced the planned closing of a second
hospital, DeWitt State, citing the age of the facility, its high per capita
patient costs, and its relatively narrow treatment program. Again the
state met with objections from the community but, in time, the state
offered the facility and its buildings to the community to be used for
schools and recreation facilities. Again the hospital was closed without
a major setback to the economy. Most employees found jobs—though
at some distance in this case—and the patients were relocated to
"board-and-care" facilities. Other events followed quickly. The state
closed Agnew State Hospital in 1971, and plans were announced to
close Mendicino State Hospital. At this point, the argument emerged
that, unlike Agnew's catchment area where Santa Clara and San Mateo
counties had effective community mental health programs, the Mendicino service area was weak in community programs. The board-and-
care facilities were declared substandard by a report of Solano County,
which was served by Napa State Hospital. Local newspapers printed
damaging editorials, especially when a former mental patient of the
state hospital shot at pedestrians. Hospital unions joined the outcry.

Faced with strong opposition, the governor announced in 1974 that no more closings would take place. More important, the California legislature, in special session, voted itself the authority to review, veto, or close any mental hospital in the future, thereby limiting the governor's power to control future hospital closings.

Similar and simultaneous efforts to close hospitals were on the way in other states. Some were more concerned about providing alternative care facilities before the closure than others. In 1971 Massachusetts announced the closure of Grafton State Hospital. Executed as an economy measure, the closing resulted in the transfer of most of the 800 patients of Grafton State Hospital to other nearby institutions. An innovation was introduced in the relocation of patients. Transfer was made in two stages. At first, the patients who could be absorbed in nearby institutions without additional staff were moved. In the second stage, where additional staff was necessary for reducing the burden of the existing staff of the receiving institution, the Grafton staff went with the patients.

In Ohio, the Cleveland State Hospital was closed as a part of a comprehensive regional plan. The state hired an energetic hospital administrator just to close the hospital. Four hundred patients were transferred to other institutions, and 300 were placed in the community. To prepare the patients for community living, halfway-house facilities were made available. Aftercare resources were identified and tapped. A community rehabilitation unit at Cleveland State Hospital worked full time to resolve community care issues.

The major issue in deinstitutionalization has not been the relocation of patients to similar facilities but whether communities can readily absorb the patients. A majority of those studying deinstitutionalization agree about the potential for normalization through active involvement in community life, but they disagree on the question of whether the health care, financial assistance, and recreational and vocational services available in certain communities are adequate to meet the needs. At issue also is whether local communities have the capacity to coordinate the support services that ex-patients need in the community. To address this issue, Virginia developed a pilot project named Service Integration and Deinstitutionalization (SID). Coordination is to be achieved through five mechanisms: assessment and prescription teams (A&P), broker advocates, quality control staff, automated information systems, and a committee of commissioners. In the pilot project, A&P teams identified services that would be helpful before, during, and after discharge, and broker advocates attempted to fill the prescriptions. The concept of broker advocates brought a measure of service integration but not new facilities. The A&P team concept defined the need, but again did not promote the building of new facilities.

In other states, the push towards closings moves ahead. In Michigan, the Macomb-Oakland Regional Center (MORC) has started major work on community placement. In the state of Pennsylvania, the Chester County MH/MR office adopted Virginia's A&P model. Other centers in other states are doing innovative placement work. Thus the major issue of where to place the patient is now being faced some six years after the first hospital closed its doors in California./

The arguments for and against hospital closings abound. They range from the fear of using untried methods to advocacy for changing the definition of the state hospital. Those who argue against closing in essence say that hospitals should not be closed for the following reasons:

1. Custodial care will always be required for some patients.
2. No alternative care facilities in the community are available. And, even if some facilities are available, the community is not ready to receive former mental patients.
3. Patients in mental hospitals require aftercare in halfway houses before being transferred to the community. Very few such facilities are available. The board-and-care facilities in the community are third-rate and are no substitute for the state hospital.
4. The massive dislocation of staff and communities where hospitals are a major industry far outweighs the advantages of relocating the patients.

Those who are for closing state hospitals give equally cogent and strong arguments:

1. The appalling conditions in state hospitals and the lack of treatment require no further justification in support of closings. If they are half as bad as they have been described, all of them should be closed.
2. If the CCMHC concept is ever going to be a way of life in America, it will require political pressure to build community care facilities. There is no better way of generating pressure for new facilities and staff than to have patients in communities who need care.
3. Whatever care the former hospital patients can get in the community is better than no care at all in a mental hospital.
4. Better service coordination with welfare agencies and other charitable groups is possible if mental patients reside in the community. All such groups ignore the mental patients once they are admitted to hospitals.

These are some of the arguments, in laymen's language, for and against closing. None of these arguments is insubstantial, but proponents of each viewpoint make it a cornerstone of the policy they advocate. Coupled with documented case histories, they make powerful statements of position. The aim of the present work, therefore, is to present all sides of the issue.

The editors have been deeply involved in the issue and bring varied, complementary backgrounds to it. The senior editor's experience in the mental health field as a program evaluator, researcher, lawyer, and economist led to his involvement in the research on the rights of patients, on the economic impact of closings on the communities, and on cost–benefit analyses of various mental health programs. The junior editor's long involvement in the mental health area as a clinical psychologist and as an author in the field prompted him to investigate the clinical aspects of the impact of mental hospital phaseouts. In an attempt to combine their experiences, the editors have produced a book dealing with economic, administrative, social, psychological, and clinical aspects arising from the closing of such hospitals. The authors presenting their works here represent a variety of backgrounds: six are psychiatrists, three sociologists, two psychologists, two economists, and one a social worker.

This book is organized in three sections. The first section presents an overall view of the social, economic, and legal forces that have affected the state hospital closings along with the arguments for and against the continuation of state-run mental hospitals. This section describes the impact of new tranquilizing drugs and the CMHC legislation on the development of mental institutions. The authors of individual chapters were selected for their leadership and considerable published work in the mental health field over many years. The expertise of Milton Greenblatt, former commissioner of mental health of Massachusetts, and now professor of psychiatry at UCLA, was sought to trace the historical forces affecting the closings of state mental hospitals and the alternatives to them. Dr. Werner Mendel of UCLA, Dr. Paul Dingman of Colgate University, and Dr. Steve Rachlin of Meyer-Manhattan Hospital were requested to write papers for and against the closures. In addition, Dr. Rachlin did a survey of the literature relating to the closings.

The second section focuses on research undertaken in the field to investigate the effects of state hospital closings. Summaries of research on the impact of the closings in New York, Massachusetts, California, and Canada have been included in this section. The chapters deal not only with the effects of relocation on patients but also with the effects of closure on hospital staff and on the communities in which hospitals have been relocated. Authors who had finished impact analysis work based on methodologically sound surveys were invited to submit papers for this section. Sam Weiner's major work on the closing of DeWitt State Hospital was included here.* Dr. E. W. Markson's study on the relocation of patients in New York and Dr. S. P. Segal's work on board and care facilities in California were also solicited for inclusion in this section. Similarly, Dr. R. Marlowe's study on the relocation of Modesto State Hospital patients is also presented. In selecting these authors and their papers, the editors included only those researches that were based on systematic surveys rather than on anecdotes or opinions.

The third section deals with some viable alternatives to state hospitals as well as with some of the services associated with the alternatives. One chapter examines the legal rights of the patients. The editors invited Prof. J. Robitscher of Emory University, who has had experience in law and psychiatry, to write an analysis of the impact of the various Supreme Court decisions on the rights of mental patients. Dr. Hugh G. Lafave's experience with the closing of the hospital in Saskatchewan deals with the issues of community care. The senior editor's article in this section looks toward the future and analyzes long-term trends in the development of mental health facilities.

This book obviously does not settle all questions relating to the closing of state hospitals or to the legal rights of the patients. Unfortunately, too many questions on the impact on patients are unanswered because of lack of support money for the development of the methodology to evaluate the impact. Follow-up of patients for such evaluation is expensive, and the impact of relocation as a single variable is hard to isolate. Similarly, even in the Donaldson decision, the Supreme Court left too many questions unanswered concerning the rights of the patients. The Court's holding that "a state cannot . . . confine without more" essentially refers to what a state cannot do, but not to what it should do. The precise definition of "more" is left for future litigation and could mean any or all of the following: adequacy of treatment, efficacy of treatment, right to treatment, aftercare, right to refuse treatment. It is hoped that many of the unanswered questions will be dealt with in other studies and books. The editors plan to treat major issues of community care in the future books of the series Current Issues in Mental Health.

---

*This study has also been reported in an article by Weiner, Place, and Ahmed in the July 1974 issue of *Administration in Mental Health.*

# 2

# Historical Factors Affecting the Closing of State Hospitals

## MILTON GREENBLATT

"The Saskatchewan Hospital, Weyburn, is no more."[1] Thus wrote Lafave and Grunberg of the dramatic closing in 1971 of the principal mental institution of southern Saskatchewan—just 50 years after it opened. It was the only psychiatric resource for a population of 500,000 in a 4,000-square-mile territory. In 1930 a small 20-bed unit was constructed in the general hospital in neighboring Regina; later 1,000 mentally retarded were transferred from Weyburn to a new facility. The 1950s brought a further decline in Weyburn's population due to the use of tranquilizers and to an enlightened administration that transformed the hospital from a custodial to a therapeutic institution. In 1956 a 24-bed unit was established in a general hospital in Moose Jaw, another adjacent territory formerly served entirely by Weyburn. In the early 1960s, five defined service areas assumed *total responsibility* for psychiatric services in their area. By 1965, with the dramatic drop in admissions and with an increasing number of discharged patients being absorbed into the regional community program, it became clear that the hospital could be closed.

And in 1971 the Weyburn hospital did close.

In America, the number of hospital closings is still small, as shown in Table I.

MILTON GREENBLATT • Veterans Administration Hospital, Sepulveda, California 91343.

Table I.   State Mental Hospital Closings in the United
States[a]

| State | Number closed | Year closed |
|-------|---------------|-------------|
| California | 1 | 1970 |
| | 3 | 1972 |
| Illinois | 1 | 1973 |
| Kentucky | 1[b] | 1971 |
| Massachusetts | 1 | 1973 |
| Minnesota | 1[c] | 1971 |
| | 1[c] | 1972 |
| New York | 1 | 1972 |
| Oklahoma | 1 | 1970 |
| | 1 | 1971 |
| Washington | 1 | 1973 |
| Wisconsin | 1 | 1973 |
| Total | 14 | |

[a]Data based on survey conducted through questionnaires distributed by
Harry C. Schnibbe and Robert Krienmyer of National Association of
State Mental Health Program Directors, October 1973.
[b]State school for the retarded.
[c]Adolescent unit.

However, because of the remarkable reduction of population and
the multiplication of community resources, we can look forward either
to a major metamorphosis in the functions of state mental hospitals or
to further total shutdowns.

We are at a point where administrators are asking themselves:
Have we waited too long? What facilities should we be phasing out
right now? What should we do to provide more adequate community
options for discharged patients? And, of course, if we phase out, what
problems do we meet?

The 50 years of Weyburn's history is a convenient span of time for
tracing the forces that have contributed to the closing of mental hospitals. We have witnessed during that period a series of remarkable
changes: from *custody* as the essential motif of care, with its punitive
and restrictive methods—such as seclusion, wet sheet packs, continuous tubs, chemical and physical restraints—to *therapy*, with its emphasis on freeing the inner person through understanding, communication, and self-realization.

A further development has taken the form of the *therapeutic community*, which in its best expressions has attempted to mobilize the
therapeutic potential of both patients and staff. The breaking down of
barriers between staff and patient and the utilization by leadership of

the principle of progressive expectations as the catalyst for a better life for all the hospital citizens have been the major elements in this development.

The transition from custody to therapy was, of course, favored by the evolution of somatic treatments—especially electric shock treatments—and the use of insulin and lobotomies. We tend to forget the excitement among therapists that attended the introduction of shock treatments, especially EST, and the enormous stimulation of morale and self-esteem among psychiatrists who felt that now at last we had a valuable therapeutic tool. Although insulin therapy was rather dangerous, nevertheless, remarkable improvement was noted in many patients with this technique. Little matter that improvements proved to be due more to concentrated personal attention than to hypoglycemia— at least *some* patients with schizophrenia were getting well.

As for lobotomy, there is no question about its being a powerful tool for changing behavior that allowed many chronic patients to be discharged to the community. What mattered most, it seemed, was the demonstration that patients formerly regarded as hopeless possessed substantial potential for improvement; this, in turn, challenged proponents of all other therapies to show what they could do for the long-term case.

The development of the concept of the therapeutic community signaled the collaboration of mental health with social science and more or less ushered in the era of social psychiatry, which, in its various manifestations, will probably dominate the rest of this century. The phaseout of hospitals is but one of the dramatic developments in this field.

The next change for the mental hospital was in the direction of the establishment of the *mental health center*. As we experienced this at Massachusetts Mental Health Center in the 1940s and 1950s, it meant open doors, early discharge, day care and transitional facilities, community volunteers, citizen education, and citizen participation. The key to this period was the breaking down of barriers between hospital and community.

Finally, in the 1960s, the mental hospital system of the nation began to move in the direction of small *comprehensive community mental health centers*. This seems to me to have come about because of a simple but significant event: the adoption by the mental hospital of responsibility for a geographically defined (catchment) area. Inevitably, there followed outreach programs, bridging services to community satellites, joint planning by hospital with community boards and service agencies for a total mental health and retardation delivery system, the burgeoning of home treatment, family and network therapies, the identification of risk groups, and preventive intervention in those risk groups.

It is hardly fair to mention the community thrust without alluding to at least one highlight: Had not Rosemary Kennedy been retarded, her family would not have suffered those peculiar torments which led them from hiding her as a family secret to openly proclaiming the cross they had to bear, and to publicly dedicating themselves to the cause of the afflicted. Fortunately for the mentally ill and retarded, John F. Kennedy supported mental health and retardation programs as they had never been supported before—or since.

As the result of historic federal initiatives, the country was given the Joint Commission on Mental Health and Illness (with American Psychiatric Association assistance), money for planning, the Community Mental Health Centers Act, funds for construction and subsequently for staffing of about 400 comprehensive community mental health centers (CCMHCs) across the nation, and the much weaker but very effective Hospital Improvement Program.

We received an expanded National Institute of Mental Health, greater emphasis on retardation, children's disorders, and eventually, drug addiction and alcoholic disorders. We also obtained rehabilitation services without discrimination as between physical and mental rehabilitation and, finally, we received strong directives toward citizen participation and consumer representation in what soon became Comprehensive Health Planning. At the same time, on the state level, money was pouring out of generous coffers to try to make something good out of mental hospitals and schools for the retarded, and thousands of citizen groups together developed a public lobby of unprecedented strength.

An illustration from personal experience: As commissioner of mental health in Massachusetts, I had to deal not only with boards of trustees for every hospital, but also with citizen boards on mental health and retardation for every one of the 39 areas in the commonwealth. In addition, there were upwards of 30 mental health associations, 30 retardation associations, plus associations for mentally ill children and, of course, numerous auxiliary and friends' associations of hospitals, clinics, and community homes. In addition to the executive branch and 280 legislators, the commissioner was beholden to about 200 citizen organizations and the families of 70,000 patients. Include also about 20,000 volunteers who not infrequently reported on sorry conditions they observed within our hospitals and clinics.

This massive citizen army will eventually prevail, we hope, in the fight for the mentally ill and retarded, and they will close many more hospitals if, indeed, that is what they think is proper in the long run.

The state legislatures and the courts certainly have played an important role. Many of the states have developed new legislation enabling their departments of mental health to go ahead with the construction and staffing of comprehensive community mental health centers. Many states have fostered local initiative by generous state matching of local contributions. Citizen groups, by law, have been given a greater voice in the planning and administration of mental health facilities. But by far the most important impact has been from those laws that have guaranteed wider rights and privileges to inmates of mental institutions, for example, the right to seek legal counsel, to communicate with friends and relatives, to have letters sent unopened to the governor and commissioner, to manage their own affairs, to hold an occupational or vehicular license, to make a will, to marry, to keep and spend a reasonable amount of money, to be admitted on a voluntary basis, if at all possible, and to terminate that admission at will.

The significance of all this is that if the patient through hospitalization is not disfranchised and can remain in communication with his group, he cannot be isolated or sequestered. Indeed, increasingly in the state laws, when retention of the patient beyond a specific time is contemplated, the burden is placed upon the superintendent to prove before the courts that this is, indeed, necessary. Periodic reviews are mandated before the patient can be considered for retention at all.

Contributing to the factors affecting patients' status in hospitals are recent court rulings at the federal and state level—pertaining to the right to adequate and appropriate treatment—first pronounced by Judge Bazelon in *Rouse* v. *Cameron*, then greatly elaborated in decisions defining the standards for adequate and appropriate treatment. The most famous of these is, of course, the ruling by Judge Johnson of the Federal Court in Alabama, whose prescription of standards for adequate and appropriate treatment, if supported by the Supreme bench, would perpetrate a veritable revolution in institutional care.

Beyond this are judgments guaranteeing educational advantages to inmates of hospitals and state schools. There are also rulings requiring that patients be paid for work done that contributes to the operation of the hospital—an end to institutional peonage.

Much of this legal advance, it should be mentioned, comes from the discovery by citizens of the class action vehicle of redress, which potentially gives the citizen advocate great power and can force upon the states huge expenditures. Small wonder, therefore, that some states are so actively seeking ways to do the job at lower cost. Obviously, treating patients earlier in their clinical course, closer to home, without disruption of work, family, or community ties, is not only more economical but immensely more humane. Why, then, be tied to institutional care with its large overhead, its artificiality, its impersonality, and relatively poor results? In a sense, our backs are to the wall; it's *phase out* before we go *bankrupt*.

These wide-ranging developments in social psychiatry, plus advances in psychopharmacology, set the stage for rapid decline in institutional population and the emergence of a veritable diaspora of community alternatives.

A typical example: The height of the population at Boston State Hospital was in 1957, when the inpatient census stood at 3,300. By the time of my superintendency, 1963 to 1967, the population had fallen to 2,400. We had a small outpatient department, a day hospital, a home treatment service, and precious little in the way of aftercare. Between 1963 and 1967, the population fell to 1,400; and in the superintendency of Dr. Jonathan Cole, 1967 to 1973, the population fell to 650. Concomitantly, the outpatient department, day hospital, aftercare, halfway houses, cooperative apartments, and home treatment increased vastly. By 1973, there were about 10 times as many patients in various forms of extramural care as there were in intramural care.

This trend was accelerated statewide during the years of my commissionership. For example, in 1967, there were approximately 150 facilities and services of the Department of Mental Health. Five years later, in January, 1972, there were more than 560. Table II shows more specific areas of expansion.

These results are not unique; similar changes are taking place in many other states in the Union. As regards reduction, in our 5-year

Table II.   Expansion of Community Programs in
Massachusetts

|                                                      | 1967   | 1972 |
|------------------------------------------------------|--------|------|
| Mental health centers                                | 2      | 15   |
| Mental health clinics                                | 37     | 57   |
| Day care programs                                    | ca. 10 | 45   |
| Community clinical nursery schools for the retarded  | 59     | 101  |
| Drug programs                                        | 6      | 155  |
| Community residences                                 | 5      | 20   |
| Court clinics                                        | 15     | 27   |

report to the governor[2] we pointed to the fact that the census in state hospitals dropped from 18,433 to 10,626 in the 9-year period from 1962 to 1971.

We noted that despite census reduction, more people were served in state hospitals—11,638 in 1962 as compared to 14,237 in 1971. But the numbers of patients cared for in the overall system rose much more dramatically as a result of the numerous community facilities, from about 25,000 to well over 70,000.

In thinking about historic forces leading to census reduction in mental hospitals, it is well to remember that major shifts had been taking place in philosophy and concepts of management. The new superintendent no longer feared the community but thought that the community might be very therapeutic for many of his patients. Not only was he more easily convinced his patients could be discharged, but when community resistance arose due to the disturbed behavior of his clients, he was willing to deal directly with the citizens, to ask their indulgence, forbearance, and further cooperation.

The new, good superintendent was interested in a variety of changes: He abhorred excessive use of seclusion; he saw great advantages to bringing men and women together in social activities and in housing facilities that could appropriately and properly accommodate both; he promoted work rehabilitation and developed paid work programs; he implemented "community preparation" wards where social skills were taught or developed; he got behind patient government on every ward—intramurally—and fostered social therapeutic clubs—extramurally; he helped establish psychiatric wards and outpatient activities in local general hospitals; he encouraged volunteers and paraprofessionals to come into the hospital to serve patients and to take them out of the hospital; he made affiliative arrangements with medical schools and other institutions of higher learning; and he invited students from *every* discipline to work and study at his hospital. Moreover, wherever he could, he developed hospital-based research and educational activities in order to create a vital and exciting intellectual climate.

Census reduction and changes in philosophy of management were accompanied by great institutional changes, the chief of which was unitization, or the decentralization of the institution into semiautonomous units, and each unit assigned responsibility for a defined catchment area. Thus, the hospital wards began to face outward; the ward plus its community became the planning base for services, and the citizens of the catchment area could become true partners to the professional staff.

The following good results flowed from unitization of hospitals:

1. Institutional change, often by itself better than no change.
2. Opportunity for formation of more responsible clinical teams; opportunity for more people to rise to leadership.
3. Greater continuity of care; patients admitted, treated, discharged, and followed up by same team.
4. Reduction of the gulf between acute and chronic patients.
5. Greater emphasis on discharge, and an *acceleration in the decrease of hospital census.*
6. Emphasis on development of day hospital and transitional facilities; home visits.
7. Formation of more citizen groups supporting the hospitals.

Historically, the roots of the phaseout of mental hospitals, therefore, go very deep—and as we move out of each phase into the next, the inevitability of a community-based system to replace the old hospital-based system becomes ever more apparent.

Let us now deal with the more immediate forces favoring closing of mental hospitals and, also, some of the forces opposing it, for both sets of forces may be operative in any event.

Some factors favoring phaseout of mental hospitals:[3]

1. Early preparation, participation, and cooperation of legislators, patients, families, labor groups, and employees.
2. *Determination* of legislators, administrators, and appropriate citizen groups to phase out.
3. Negligible disruption of the community's economy.
4. Sharp reduction in hospital population as function of success of hospital treatment program in discharging patients and availability of community placements and options, i.e., community mental health centers, clinics, etc.
5. Reduced admissions to the hospital as a function of increased admissions to other facilities and services, such as (a) psychiatric units in general hospitals, (b) small new community mental health centers, (c) satellite clinics and aftercare services, or (d) administrative assignment of hospital's catchment area to another facility.
6. High per-patient costs for inpatient service, especially as a result of reduced census, and high administrative overhead—in contrast to low per-patient costs for service in the community.
7. Intolerably poor quality of inpatient care.

8. Outmoded, inadequate, or condemned physical plants, too costly to renovate or replace.
9. Availability of other inpatient facilities for direct transfer of patients.
10. Guarantee of job security for every employee at same level of pay, with appropriate seniority rights, and with negligible personal sacrifice in terms of family dislocation, commuting, and living conditions in the community of relocation.
11. Job retraining for those moved into new positions without cost to the employee.
12. Positive use of abandoned plant and facilities.
13. Demonstration that patients fare better under the new conditions, are not an excessive burden on the welfare rolls, and do not disrupt unduly the equanimity of the community because of untoward behavior.

Forces opposing or retarding the phaseout of mental hospitals would include the following:

1. Inadequate education or cooperation of executive and legislative arms of government or out-and-out opposition by either of these branches.

2. Battle between the legislative and executive branch, usually the executive favoring and the legislative opposing phaseout, an especially heated struggle if the two branches are of opposing political parties.

3. Resistance of hospital personnel—superintendent or staff. Usually this takes the form of superintendent's anxiety about his future and a feeling that as his hospital diminishes in size, so does he diminish in professional and personal stature. Also, there is great reluctance to presiding over a dying organization, and it is progressively more difficult to carry on in the presence of decaying morale.[4] Important assistants and staff may jump the gun, finding jobs elsewhere as the psychological and administrative burden of phasedown threatens. Complaints, accusations, and tensions are likely to mount during critical periods. Since the hospital selected for phaseout is often one whose program has lagged or where patient care has been less than satisfactory, the phaseout may be viewed as public notice of failure of the hospital's administration.

Resistance may come not only from personnel employed in the institution to be closed but also from the institution which may receive the patients in transfer. The latter institution may see it all as a bad bargain. They may resent receiving chronic patients with low rehabilitation potential, particularly if no new staff personnel are added.

It is obvious that the greatest care must be taken in preparing all parties to the transfer, so that morale, the sine qua non for good patient treatment, is maintained.

4. Resistance of patients and families. The threat of a phaseout raises everyone's anxieties. Rumor and gossip multiply fantasies. Patients may react with deepening illness. (The threat of phasing out one building of 80 chronic female patients at Boston State Hospital was accompanied by one acute coronary and one acute cerebral vascular accident. We strongly suspected psychosomatic reaction to the threat of impending disaster.)

Relatives instinctively fear transfer trauma[5] and the breakup of stable relationships. Staff and patients have developed long-standing mutual support systems. Elderly patients are known to be at risk of early demise, especially when the separation is viewed by them as a decline in the quality of their life, or as a terminal placement.

On the other hand, if the patient is to be moved into the community, the family may fear that the patient will come home to them—revisiting upon them burdens they had long since shifted to the state. Parents of retarded youngsters may resist their placement in the community with the same vigor that they fought for upgrading of care and treatment within the institution.

5. Resistance from labor. Labor will be concerned about protection of jobs, and rights and privileges—especially seniority rights, conditions of work, and special hardship to their members. Workers will be concerned about costs of relocation, commuting distance, loss of second jobs for themselves or other family members, schooling of children, and disruption of friendship patterns in their community. The fragile truce between labor and the establishment can be easily broken by a few bad moves, the worst of which is not to bring labor leaders into planning before union members start peppering them with complaints and exaggerated rumors.

6. Resistance from the community. This takes several forms. One is concern about the release of "unattractive" and "misbehaving" patients into the community, lowering the quality of life, so to speak. Robert Reich and Lloyd Siegel[6] have written dramatically of the neglect and suffering of chronic patients released from New York hospitals as part of their phasedown. Their derelict existence rivals that of the chronic alcoholic. They burden the welfare rolls, crowd flophouses, sleep in subways. The authors raise the disturbing question as to what has been gained by moving these patients from the protection of the ward to the oblivion of the gutter.

A second concern arises if plans are developing for establishment of community homes, cooperative apartments, halfway houses, rehabilitation workshops, or geriatric centers, especially in middle- or upper-class neighborhoods, where residents feel they have finally achieved some sense of gracious, genteel, quiet, dignified living—away from the madding world. Try to open a halfway house in some of these neighborhoods, especially if there is no guarantee against drugs and alcoholism.

A third concern arises from the business community, the small shopkeepers, the motel and guest house proprietors, the food market managers who have been dependent upon trade from the hospital and its staff. The outcry will be proportional to the degree of dependence of that community upon hospital business. Unfortunately, this can be very considerable, especially when hospitals are situated in small towns, or when the economic life of an area is marginal. If, however, a compensatory future is planned for the institution—such as a school, a nursing home, a work camp—the business community may be mollified (as in the case of Saskatchewan). Without such conversion, the institution stands as an empty shell, a prey to vandalism.

It is obvious that these forces, pro and con the closing of mental hospitals, are shaped both qualitatively and quantitatively by their history and their own particular conditions. If the hospital has a shining image as a place of quality care and a home of refuge for the distressed, the staff and the citizens are likely to bristle at any plans to close it. If the hospital has a snake-pit reputation, fewer will be willing to keep it alive. If community resources have been cultivated, if the population decline is well known, and the community-based philosophy is accepted, that hospital will have less difficulty phasing out.

What lies ahead may well be heralded by the headline in *Psychiatric News* of December 19, 1973, "California Shelves Plans for Abolishing Hospitals."[7]

> The Reagan administration had planned to phase out all California state mental hospitals by 1982, but now plans to keep 11 institutions in operation for the time being. They will take on expanded functions in care for a wide variety of patients, ranging from mentally disturbed sex offenders to retarded children. A network of treatment facilities for violent patients has also been proposed.
>
> The administration's plans to phase out state hospitals had been announced against a backdrop of increasing public alarm over a series of murders and other violent crimes by persons who had been treated as mental patients. Parents of hospitalized mentally retarded children had protested the phase out. . . . Democratic gubernatorial contenders accused the Governor of "dumping" patients into communities unprepared to care for them. . . .

This announcement was soon followed by a headline story in the *Los Angeles Times*[8] that Governor Reagan's veto of a bill requiring

legislative approval before any state institution could be phased out
had been overridden by the legislature. This was historically significant, for such an override had not occurred in 28 years of California
political history.

It is most significant that the state which has taken the most
vigorous leadership in phasing out institutions should have that trend
suddenly put under control of the legislature taking into its hands
powers traditionally reserved to the executive branch. Is it part of a
broad national trend toward increasing legislative control of health and
health research? We think so.

Will other state legislatures follow? Will this mean that mental
institutions will become more of a political football than they are now?
Or is it all part of an awakened public consciousness of the work to be
done on behalf of the mentally ill with greater participation and responsibility in this task by the representatives of the people?

## References

1. Lafave, H. G., & Grunberg, F. *La Fin de l'asile* 1976 (in press).
2. Greenblatt, M., Commissioner, Massachusetts Department of Mental Health. *Challenge and response: A five-year progress report on the Comprehensive Mental Health and Retardation Services Act of the Commonwealth of Massachusetts, January 1973.*
3. Weiner, S., Bird, B. J., & Bolton A., Associates. *Process and impacts of the closing of DeWitt State Hospital: Final report, May 1973.* Funded under Grant No. MH 19222-01, 02, Division of Mental Health Services Program, Office of Program Planning and Evaluation, NIMH, U.S. Department of HEW, SRI Project URU-1147. Menlo Park, California: Stanford Research Institute.
4. Stotland, E., & Kobler, A. L. *Life and death of a mental hospital.* Seattle: University of Washington Press, 1965.
5. Greenblatt, M. Therapeutic and non-therapeutic features of the environment. In M. Greenblatt, M. H. Solomon, A. S. Evans, & G. W. Brooks (Eds.), *Drug and social therapy in chronic schizophrenia.* Springfield, Illinois: Charles C Thomas, 1965. Pp. 214–217.
6. Reich, R., & Siegel, L. Psychiatry under siege: The chronic mentally ill shuffle to oblivion. *Psychiatric Annals,* November 1973, **3,** 35–55.
7. California shelves plans for abolishing hospitals. *Psychiatric News,* December 19, 1973, **24,** 1.
8. Endicott, W. Reagan overridden on veto first time. *Los Angeles Times,* January 29, 1974, p. 1.

# 3

# The Case for Closing of the Hospitals

WERNER M. MENDEL

The hospital as a form of treatment for the severely ill psychiatric patient is always expensive and inefficient, frequently antitherapeutic, and never the treatment of choice.

There are many studies in the psychiatric literature of the last two decades which report that forms of treatment other than hospitalization are superior in terms of outcome for the severely ill psychiatric patient.[1,2,3,4] These studies were conducted in a variety of centers across the American continent and Europe and each produced similar results. In terms of the patients' posttreatment function, need for further treatment, and improvement in symptoms, patients who were not hospitalized always did better than matched patients who were treated in hospitals. Those individuals whose severe psychiatric illnesses were treated in home settings, day care, night shelters, outpatient clinics, or by crisis teams had far better treatment results. Such findings are now so reliably demonstrated in many centers that they are no longer surprising.

Even prior to the past two decades it had been well established that prolonged hospitalization was always antitherapeutic.[5,6,7] Much of what had been described as the final outcome of chronic mental illness

WERNER M. MENDEL • University of Southern California School of Medicine, Los Angeles, California 90033.

turned out to be the outcome of chronic hospitalization. Logically, it makes little sense to hospitalize someone because he has problems with feelings, thoughts, or behavior. It makes even less sense to add to the patient's dysfunction the special problem of having to live and adjust to the complex society of a collection of psychiatric patients and peculiar staff in a strange setting and with multiple and complex agendas. Even for those of us who are relatively free of severe illness, dealing with the formal and informal structure and agenda in a psychiatric ward requires all our sensitivity and adaptive capacity. Think then what an illogical and impossible requirement it is to ask such adaptation from a mental patient who by definition has problems with behavior, feelings, and thoughts.

The decision to hospitalize an individual is not based on the treatment needs of the patient nearly as much as on the needs of society, the family, and the treating physician.[8,9] Even when the decision-maker believes he is making the decision to hospitalize on a clinical basis, the decision is made, in fact, on the basis of social, economic, and professional habits. In our study of hospital admissions, the patients hospitalized are clinically indistinguishable from those not hospitalized even when the decision to use the hospital is made by senior, experienced clinicians.

If we look at the reasons for which hospitalization has been prescribed in the past, it becomes clear[10] that each and every one of these functions can be better and much less expensively carried out, and with fewer negative side effects, in settings other than a psychiatric hospital ward.

Let us look at those functions which we traditionally carry out in the hospital, all of which can be better carried out in alternative settings when these are available. These alternatives include day treatment, group living, patient sitters, peer-group support, and crisis teams.[11]

1. Is the patient's present condition so disturbed that he is unable to maintain the relationship with the therapist that is necessary for outpatient management during the period of exacerbation? Here, such factors must be considered as: his ability to keep appointments, his level of functioning, his ability to care for his social and biological needs, his capacity to mobilize enough aid from significant others to have his needs met.

2. Is the patient's impulse control so tenuous that he and other significant figures in his life are too fearful to tolerate attempts to manage an exacerbation on an outpatient basis? If so, intensive care is necessary in order to demonstrate control and thus to relieve the patient of this anxiety.

3. Has the patient by his disturbed behavior alienated himself from the organizing and supportive resources formerly available to him, such as his job, his family, community agencies? When these resources withdraw their support because they are no longer willing to tolerate his disturbance and his demands, then the homeostasis is quickly upset and the patient is in need of finding other support to which his disturbed behavior is more acceptable. One such support, of course, is the hospital. This very reason for hospitalization, however, is also one of the important disadvantages of hospital treatment. In general, unless very carefully supervised, hospitals tend to reinforce and support sick behavior rather than healthy behavior, and to that extent they tend to be antitherapeutic. On occasion brief hospitalization (by brief hospitalization I mean several days of hospitalization) may prevent a permanent alienation of the helping resources that were formerly mobilized by the patient. However, a successful alternative to hospitalization is the "crash pad" or motel in conjunction with day care and crisis intervention.

4. Has the patient used pathological behavior in an attempt to cope with his exacerbation (excessive use of alcohol or drugs, malnutrition, exhaustion) to such an extent that treatment is now necessary to correct secondary problems?

5. Has there been a loss of a major source of support, through death or other circumstances not brought about by the patient? In considering this indication for crisis care, hospitalization is the least desirable alternative.

6. Does the patient need to be protected from self-destruction or from hurting others? This use of hospitalization is traditional. When a patient cannot be prevented from committing suicide or from inflicting harm on others, some technique of massive crisis intervention is necessary as a measure of control. There are other and better methods of preventing a patient from committing suicide than placing him in hospital. The potential danger to others is frequently overestimated by the therapist. These are always difficult decisions to make and must be based on careful consideration of the patient's history of impulse control, the number of supporting and controlling factors available to him in the environment, the readiness with which he is able to use a human relationship as a helping situation, and the chronicity of the danger of self-destruction or of hurting others.

7. Is the patient in need of being protected from the possible consequences of his actions? A patient who, during exacerbation of illness or during psychotic episodes, behaves in a way that will in the future change his life situation may require crisis intervention briefly.

A patient who during an exacerbation behaves in business in such a way that he will lose his customers or dissipate his resources should be protected from his actions. A patient who endangers his associations, friendships, business contacts, and professional relationships during a brief period of exacerbation might well be removed from his customary psychosocial life space to prevent the rupture of these relationships.

8. Does the patient need crisis care at this time in the management of his illness to reinforce the therapeutic intent? On occasion, especially at the beginning of treatment, it is necessary to offer intensive care to a patient in order to establish the relationship with the helping situation and to establish the patient's role.

9. Do the regularly available supportive resources need a brief vacation from the patient? This approach to the use of hospitalization has been successfully used in England in the care of geriatric patients. There are many families who can tolerate a very sick member in their midst if they are given the opportunity for occasional vacations. In the long-term management of such patients, it seems to me that an appropriate indication for alternate placement away from their home includes allowing the supportive resources the opportunity to gather new strengths to deal with the patient.

10. Is the patient in need of training in healthy behavior? Many chronic patients need help in adopting a new "as if" role in which a more adaptive facade is developed. On occasion the hospital has been a satisfactory place in which to retrain patients in healthy behavior, although this retraining function is best carried out in the community in which the patient lives by intensive contact between the patient and the therapist in the patient's own life space.

11. Is the patient in need of the interruption of his isolation? The increasing alienation from others frequently seen in chronic patients tends to snowball and to result in more serious and severe malfunctioning. The patient might sit in his room 24 hours a day, 168 hours a week. His only contact with another human being may be his 1 hour of therapy a week. When such a condition exists, it may be necessary to interrupt his isolation and to bring the patient in contact with the crisis team or into the day hospital for a brief period in order to help him establish a level of adaptive capacity by which, once again, he can reach out to others. The crisis center can juxtapose the patient to others while helping him to manage his anxiety.

12. Is the patient in need of redefinition of the sick role? Certain patients who, by their behavior, get themselves placed in other roles such as the criminal, the sinner, or the "no good" person may find it impossible to function in these roles and may need to be redefined in

the sick role. Placing an individual in the hospital clearly defines him as a sick person. Such a redefinition, which can sometimes be accomplished by no more than a few hours of hospitalization, may alter his homeostasis so markedly that behavior can become more adaptive.

13. Is the patient in need of therapeutic containment (restraint) for the management of his anxiety? This is closely related to item 2 in this list: the relief of anxiety by others taking over the controls. In the chronically psychotic patient, one of the major sources of anxiety may be the recognition of poor impulse control. The patient lives as though he were sitting on top of a volcano that is about to erupt. Coming into the crisis center and having someone else take over control of the volcano markedly lowers the anxiety level in the patient and allows for immediate improvement. All of us have seen patients who have given up their grossly disorganized behavior after a few hours of crisis treatment.

14. Is hospitalization demanded by others such as the police, the judge, or the family? If the demand for hospitalization is made by others, frequently the question can best be dealt with by supportive contact with those who are demanding hospitalization. If these others are the police or a judge, contact may be difficult to carry out. On such occasions, it may be necessary to hospitalize a patient against his will and against the will of the therapist. Most states still have systems where the judiciary is in a position of making a final and binding medical decision.

15. Is it necessary to remove the patient from a chaotic and pathogenic environment? All too frequently, this reason for hospitalization is not valid, since the therapist tends to judge the patient's environment by his own middle-class standards. We must remember that many chronic patients create their environment to meet their need for lack of closeness, lack of involvement, and reification of the internal chaos in the external circumstance. On some occasions the environment set up by the patient is such that it cannot be adaptively handled by the patient. Even under such circumstances it is best to attempt to find the necessary support and reorganization in the patient's world without removing him from it.

16. Are biological interventions planned that are better carried out in the hospital? When large doses of drugs are to be tried which may have serious side effects, treatment may be more safely carried out in the controlled environment of the hospital. Electroconvulsive treatment for emergency control of serious suicidal wishes and depression is always best administered in a hospital setting.

The negative effects of all hospitalization can be prevented by using alternate approaches to providing the 16 services listed which are traditionally housed in the package of the psychiatric hospital. These inherent antitherapeutic factors in all hospitalization are:

1. Excessive gratification of dependency wishes.
2. Reinforcement of the patient's failure in life.
3. Removal of a patient who has a tenuous hold on reality and the world around him to the totally strange and peculiar environment of the psychiatric hospital. In the hospital he utilizes his remaining feeble ego resources to adjust to a psychotic environment.
4. Removal of the patient from the world, his family, and his psychosocial space alters the social homeostasis. Frequently, removing the patient from his environment results in great difficulty for him in ever moving back into that psychosocial space where his place has been lost.
5. The secondary effects of hospitalization on the patient's life are of great consequence legally, socially, and psychologically. The patient has to live with the history of having had a psychiatric hospitalization forever after. It changes his life career. Studies have shown that the decision for future hospitalization for psychiatric difficulty is influenced by history of previous hospitalization more than any other factors.[8]

The financial expense of hospitalization is another extremely important consideration in these days of the limited funds for health care. When we recognize that the hospital requires expensive medical personnel to carry out primarily nonmedical functions, the use of bed space when beds are not the primary mode of treatment for psychiatric patients, it becomes clear that the hospital is an expensive packaging for psychiatric treatment. The concept of critical-incident costing—that is, how much it costs to attain a special goal—demonstrates clearly the folly of hospitalization.[12] When the technique of goal-attainment scaling[13] is combined with the critical-incident cost accounting, it is possible to calculate quite accurately what it costs to accomplish a specific treatment goal; i.e., to stop someone from hallucinating, to stop someone from attempting suicide, to get someone back to work, to rehabilitate someone so that he is financially self-supporting, to get an individual to the point of being able to live by himself and take care of himself, to help someone be free of specific signs and symptoms. To take a severely psychotic patient who is judged to require hospitalization and to treat him with family crisis intervention until he can function on the usual outpatient supportive basis in the community costs $960. Treating him with day care and one or two days of overnight stays in a motel costs $790. However, reaching the same treatment goal in a hospital costs from \$2,900 to \$50,400, depending on the hospital. When these two techniques are applied to comparing hospital treatment with other forms of treatment, the hospital is at least three times as expensive as nonhospital treatment and also it is less effective as measured by the best available short-term and long-term outcome studies.

We must raise the question, why do we then still hospitalize in many places? Psychiatric patients continue to be placed in hospitals even though hard data are now available, and have been for some two decades, to show that the psychiatric hospital is expensive and relatively ineffective while having many negative and antitherapeutic outcomes. The reasons for continued hospitalization seem to fall into six categories:

1. It is difficult for professionals to change their behavior, including traditional and learned treatment behavior. Much of the ritual of treatment is an institutionalized repetition compulsion which functions to alleviate the anxiety of the professional and the patient.

2. It is difficult for society to give up the traditions which are more than 500 years old. Dorothea Dix, the wild woman of mental hospital reform of the mid-19th century, built over 30 hospitals to care for the mentally ill only to find out at the end of her long life that the programs and care in the hospitals were no better than the care in the jails where she had had her first shocking exposure to mental illness.

3. Society sees hospitals as good, health-giving places even though it is aware of how much mischief is carried out in hospitals. Society seems to need talismans like hospitals, temples, health spas, etc., to ward off anxiety about illness, death, and the ambiguities of life.[14] In spite of available overwhelming evidence of the need to wash, physicians steadfastly refused to wash their hands after autopsy prior to delivering babies. Yet women persisted in going to hospitals to die of septicemia by the hundreds.

4. Alternatives to hospitalization have not been adequately developed in many parts of the world even though some alternatives have existed for centuries. Developing alternatives requires effort and funding. Effort to do things differently is hard to come by and money is scarce.

5. There are economic benefits to the therapist in collecting patients in hospitals. These include the physical convenience which allows the practitioner to see many patients in rapid succession on the ward where patients wait 168 hours per week to have 5-minute "therapy" sessions with their doctor five times each week.

6. Physicians have a tradition of not being concerned with cost efficiency of treatment. Only lately, when third-party payment and

government have forced us to look at cost containment have we become concerned. Getting the most use out of each treatment dollar has at long last become an important concern for doctor and patient alike.

## Summary

Since the hospital as a form of treatment for the severely ill psychiatric patient is always expensive and inefficient, frequently antitherapeutic, and never the treatment of choice, it behooves us now to develop a strategy and timetable for dismantling the mental hospital. This strategy must include:

1. Designing alternatives to hospitalization.
2. Retraining of health professionals.
3. Educating the public.
4. Funding for alternatives before funding for hospitals is cut off.
5. Funding new functions for the existing hospital buildings and grounds and certain personnel. (An example of the need for this is seen in the work of Hugh Lafave in Saskatchewan.[15]
6. Changing psychiatric, psychological, social work, and nursing training programs to prepare the future practitioners for new roles appropriate for nonhospital treatment of mental patients.

## References

1. Taylor, R., & Torrey, E. *Mental health coverage under a national health insurance pli n.* Unpublished paper presented at the American Psychiatric Association Meeting, May 1973.
2. Herz, M., Endicott, J., Spitzer, R., & Mesnikoff, A. Day versus inpatient hospitalization: A controlled study. *American Journal of Psychiatry*, 1971, **127**, 1371–1380.
3. Wilder, J. F., Levin, G., Zwerling, I. A two year follow-up evaluation of acute psychiatric patients treated in a day hospital. *American Journal of Psychiatry*, 1966, **122**, 1095–1101.
4. Langsley, D., Machotka, P., & Flomenhaft, K. Avoiding mental hospital admission: A follow-up study. *American Journal of Psychiatry*, 1971, **127**, 1391–1394.
5. Mendel, W. Effect of length of hospitalization on rate and quality of remission from acute psychotic episodes. *Journal of Nervous and Mental Disease*, 1966, **143**, 226–233.
6. Mendel, W. On the abolition of the psychiatric hospital. Chapter 11 in *Comprehensive mental health*. Madison: The University of Wisconsin Press, 1968, pp. 237–247.
7. Mendel, W. Brief hospitalization techniques. In J. Masserman (Ed.), *Current psychiatric therapies* (Vol. 4). New York: Grune and Stratton, 1966, pp. 310–316.
8. Mendel, W., & Rapport, S. Determinants of the decision for psychiatric hospitalization. *Archives of General Psychiatry*, 1969, **20**, 321–328.

9. Miller, S., & Riessman, F. *Social class and social policy*. New York: Basic Books, 1968, pp. 164–165.

10. Dreyfus, D. A workable alternative. In *One system—ten services. Journal of the State of California Department of Mental Hygiene*, **4**(1), 4–8, Sacramento, California, April 1973.

11. Mendel, W. Prescribing crisis treatment. Chapter 9 in *Supportive care*. Los Angeles: Mara Books, 1975, pp. 82–95.

12. Mendel, W., Rapport, S., & Glasser, J. High quality, low cost prepaid psychiatric service. *World Journal of Psychosynthesis*, October 1974, **6**(10), 24–30.

13. Kiresuk, T., & Sherman, R. Goal attainment scaling: A general method of evaluating comprehensive community mental health programs. *Community Mental Health Journal*, 1968, **4**(6), 443–453.

14. Mendel, W. *Lepers, madmen, who's next?* NIMH *Schizophrenia Bulletin*, 1975, 5–8.

15. Stewart, A., Lafave, H., Grunberg, M., & Herjanic, M. Problems in phasing out a large public psychiatric hospital. *American Journal of Psychiatry*, 1968, **125**(1), 120–126.

# 4

# The Case Against Closing of State Hospitals

STEPHEN RACHLIN

Less than a generation ago, the neuroleptic drugs were introduced into psychiatric practice. With this major advance came the hope that hundreds of thousands of chronically mentally ill individuals could lead more normal lives. The public mental hospital (a term I will use synonymously with state hospital) could finally become a place of active treatment, and the days of the so-called snake pit would be at an end. In the 1960s, it became clear that many patients could be more effectively treated outside of the hospital. The community mental health centers would, perhaps, become the locus of treatment for the majority of patients. Once again, the state hospital was in disfavor.

Steinhart[1] points out how the original theme of keeping patients at home whenever possible has become ritualized into that of keeping patients completely out of state hospitals. The community mental health center movement, he tells us, sees the hospital as being destructive at best. Black[2] considers us to be, "barreling along on the road that is taking mental health services from the state hospitals to the local communities. . . ." He cautions us to stop, look, and listen before proceeding further. But, as Fischer and Weinstein[3] note, psychiatry has always shown its readiness to board the newest bandwagon. They, too, recommend that some restraint be exercised on the way toward innovation.

STEPHEN RACHLIN • Meyer-Manhattan Psychiatric Center, New York, New York 10035.

We are now in the mid-1970s, and the reputation of the public mental hospital has changed very little. The proposed solution, for some mysterious reason, is presented not in terms of upgrading quality of service, but rather as a proposition to close most, if not all, of the state hospitals. I agree with Bennett's[4] thinking that the arguments for closing have never been clearly stated. It is my contention that we will need state hospitals for the foreseeable future, and it is this thesis which will be developed in the pages that follow.

## Who Are the Patients?

There are certain "types" of patients who seem particularly unwelcome in the newer systems of care delivery. Those with hopes of eliminating state hospitals have overlooked "the desire of mental health professionals to get rid of undesirable patients."[4]

One such group is the severely ill patients who require involuntary hospitalization. While the issues surrounding this controversy are, to a certain extent, separate and distinct from those relating to hospital closure, the overlap is considerable. My associates and I[5] have previously stated our viewpoint, holding that the right to treatment must be given precedence over that of unrestricted liberty. The American Psychiatric Association has likewise recognized the need to retain statutory provisions for involuntary hospitalization of some mentally ill people.[6]

In most communities, involuntary admission is the prevalent route to the public mental hospital. Zwerling et al.[7] found that, of 125 consecutive admissions studied, 62% were based on a two-physician certificate. These patients were not any different demographically from those admitted voluntarily, but there were significant discrepancies in presenting symptoms. The involuntary patients were more likely to be characterized as showing antisocial attitudes and acts; anger, belligerence, and negativism; agitation and hyperactivity; and assaultive acts. The state hospital has always accepted the responsibility of caring for patients with these forms of behavior.

Another category of patient who has always been within the province of the state hospital is the chronically ill individual whom Rosenblatt[8] has characterized as a "weary sojourner in a hostile world." Such a person is likely to return to the hospital repeatedly. Rosenblatt and Mayer[9] reviewed the literature and determined that the strongest predictor of rehospitalization, indeed the only variable with distinguishing value, was the number of previous admissions. This held true regardless of attendance at aftercare programs.

Talbott[10] investigated the reasons for readmission to inpatient status and studied possible means for preventing such an eventuality. He found that the majority of patients were returned to the hospital because of psychotic or paranoid behavior. Almost one-third also demonstrated aggressive or assaultive patterns. The research team was of the opinion that 84% of the patients studied might not have needed rehospitalization if appropriate services had been available elsewhere; the fact remains that they were not.

Another report documenting the failure of alternatives to hospitalization in preventing chronicity is that of Smith and associates.[11] They compared a regional center, based on the community mental health model, with the traditional state hospital, and found that neither system was successful with a small, hard-core group of long-term patients. While there were benefits in many parameters to the community-based facility, it was not superior in decreasing the disability due to serious mental disorder. It seems that the technology to prevent chronicity in all patients does not exist.

Conclusion: There are certain patients, particularly the severely ill and the chronically ill, who will somehow always be guided back to the public mental hospital.

## What Happens to the Patients?

Granted that the chronically mentally ill exist, and granted also that many of them are no longer in hospitals, let us turn our attention to how well they fare in their communities. Most such patients carry a diagnosis of schizophrenia, and this term is often used interchangeably with that of chronic mental illness.

While it is generally agreed that aftercare services need to be provided for the patient who has been discharged from the hospital, the reality remains that the results of such treatment are inconsistent. Having researched the issues, Zwerling[12] states: "A review of the literature leads compellingly to the conclusion that, even with the most effective programs devised, considerable disability may be expected in the greatest number of patients."

Hogarty, Goldberg, and their group[13] have done long-term controlled aftercare studies of drug and sociotherapy in the treatment of discharged schizophrenics. One of their measures was of the effectiveness of major role therapy and chlorpromazine, in various combinations, in forestalling relapse. They found no significant effect of sociotherapy on this parameter. At the end of one year, 67.5% of the placebo-treated patients, and 30.9% of those drug-treated, had relapsed. By the time the 2-year study was completed, the figures rose to 80% for those taking placebo, and 48% for those on active medication. Thus, almost half of the drug-treated patients relapsed within 2 years.

Medication is clearly the most important dimension in the aftercare of schizophrenic individuals. Serban and Thomas[14] undertook the measurement of the attitudes of such patients toward continuing treatment subsequent to hospital discharge and compared this with the actual utilization of such therapy. In their sample, 73.9% of the chronically schizophrenic patients, and 44.3% of the acute schizophrenics, were readmitted during the 2-year follow-up period. They found extreme noncompliance with instructions for drug use by the chronically ill sample. Of the 41.9% of such patients who reported nonuse of medication, 67.8% of these said that medication could be helpful. Only 29.3% of the total "chronic" group stated that they took medication as prescribed, and, when the researchers checked this information with patients' relatives and others, the figure dropped to a mere 19.9%. Attitudes toward professional aftercare showed the same trends. While 72.3% of the chronically ill patients claimed that such treatment would be beneficial, 44% did not seek outpatient care, 27.7% were irregular attendees, and only 28% reported consistent follow-through with treatment plans. For the chronically schizophrenic person, they conclude, nonuse of medication and lack of aftercare attendance are highly related to the probability of readmission.

Looking at those patients discharged from the hospital to the community and remaining there for 2 to 3 years, Astrachan and colleagues[15] found that virtually none was symptom free. One-quarter were actively psychotic, and over two-thirds showed some psychotic symptoms. In our own study of community adjustment,[16] patients who received approved discharges were shown to be doing better than a group of self-discharged patients (elopees), but even the former group was not functioning at a high level.

Many discharged mental patients are not really living in the community. Lamb and Goertzel[17] feel that it is an illusion to consider those individuals placed in boarding or family care homes as being in the community. Such facilities are "like small long-term state hospital wards isolated from the community." The patients are overwhelmingly dependent, show insufficient ego strength to deal with crises, and continue to have symptoms. In a 5-year follow-up of long-term patients discharged to the community, these same authors[18] found that most were not functioning well. Over two-thirds were located in institutional settings, which the authors define as including boarding homes. They provide clinical vignettes of patients who need the kinds of services which are now available only in state hospitals and conclude that there is a cadre of patients for whom placement elsewhere is unlikely and who therefore will require continuing inpatient care.

Conclusion: Even if the severely ill and the chronically ill can be considered to be in the community, they are neither thriving nor prospering.

## How Are the Patients Received?

As increasing numbers of chronically ill mental patients are returned to the community, the general population has more frequent and more direct contact with them. On the one hand, this may enhance public understanding of, and empathy with, schizophrenics. Alternatively, of course, the reverse may take place.

Rabkin[19] reminds us that the label of "patient" is given to a person who is admitted to a hospital and, in the case of psychiatric illness, the label is applied to that person for an indefinite period subsequent to release. The mentally ill are regarded with "more distaste and less sympathy than virtually any other disabled group in our society." The public rejection has been rather tenacious. Based on her review of the literature relating to attitudes, Rabkin endorses the conclusion that "a major portion of the population continues to be frightened and repelled by the notion of mental illness. Today, as in times past, when people encounter the description or presence of someone who has been labeled mentally ill, they are not pleased to meet him."

As an example of public feeling, the work of Bentz and Edgerton[20] may be cited. They found that, despite generally positive changes in perceptions of mental illness and optimism regarding treatment outcome, a significant percentage of the general public saw protection of the community as a primary role of the mental hospital. These same people, then, are asked to come into greater contact with deviance as a result of the community orientation of mental health care. As Mosher and Gunderson[21] put it, the average man in the street has experienced discomfort because of the behavior of some patients. They warned us to expect a backlash against our community efforts. This backlash did occur, and I will outline some of the forms this reaction has taken in a subsequent section of this chapter.

There is a particular group of citizens who have, perhaps, the most difficult time of it when patients do not do well outside the hospital: their families. It is the relatives who must bear the burden of patient management in the community.[22] Kreisman and Joy[23] detail how families may be hard pressed and strained by the demands of the ill member. Many are reluctant to have the patient return home, especially as the number of rehospitalizations increases. Specific case examples of the cost to the family, not only in terms of dollars, but also in terms of stress, are given by Rabiner and Lurie.[24] They question whether the avoidance of hospitalization has really produced gains.

Several authors [1,5,21] have likewise commented about the needs of the families. Modlin[25] believes that more attention needs to be paid to the rights of the family and the community, even though priority must be given to the rights of the patients. The incompatibilities, if any, between these sets of rights may be more fiction than fact. I have previously reported[26] that a closed ward is required for a small proportion of patients in a state hospital. The families and the communities welcomed this form of treatment, and the patients themselves did not find it a bad place to be. In a follow-up study,[5] we demonstrated family and community pressures for increasing utilization of the closed ward, to the point where subterfuge and misrepresentation were used in order to secure admission of patients to such a specialized treatment modality. This illustrates the depth and strength of the way in which the community in which I work (New York City) may attempt to rid itself of its troublesome mentally ill.

The irrational thinking, feeling, and behavior patterns of response by an individual or by a society to the behavior of the mentally ill has been labeled "sanism" by Birnbaum.[27] He quite properly considers this a form of bigotry. Lest this phenomenon be considered an isolated one, he gives examples of its application at various levels of society. Legislatures have perpetuated the inadequate conditions which prevail in mental hospitals by insufficient funding. Mental health professionals know this situation well, often accept it, and may press to divert funds away from the state hospital system despite obvious need. Until quite recently, courts were refusing to hear cases relating to civilly committed mentally ill patients. Birnbaum calls sanism "an American tragedy," and how right he is.

Conclusion: The community is less than overjoyed to have the severely ill and the chronically ill in its midst.

## How Does the System Operate?

A fair amount of experience has been accumulated and reported, so that the actual modus operandi of community treatment of the chronically mentally ill may be assessed. Three examples will be cited: California, New York, and Great Britain.

## California

The state of California has experienced an 80% drop in its state hospital population during the decade ending in 1973. As a result of changes in their mental health law, it has become increasingly difficult to obtain admission to state hospitals and for patients to remain therein for lengthy periods. With the more seriously ill individuals in the communities, and the hospitals not as readily available to enable the exclusion of patients, other techniques for ostracizing unwanted persons are being developed. Aviram and Segal[28] call attention to the variety of ways in which the dynamics of exclusion continue to operate. Among the methods they describe are bureaucratic maneuvering, ghettoization, restrictive zoning, and the like. Abramson[29] reports that patients are increasingly being subject to arrest so that penal code commitments may be used to secure long-term hospitalization on the grounds of incompetency to stand trial. When society has reached its level of tolerance for disordered behavior, pressure is exerted to use the criminal justice system to return patients to hospitals.

A committee of the California Senate was charged with the responsibility of investigating the proposed phaseout of state hospital services. Extensive hearings were held, and persons from all walks of life were heard. In its final report,[30] the committee confirmed problems emanating from inadequate living arrangements and neighborhoods, the inclusion of jails in the revolving-door syndrome, and the lack of adequate follow-up care. Based on the evidence presented, the committee also raised serious questions about the effectiveness of the community mental health programs with the chronically ill patients discharged from hospitals, stating that certain types of patients cannot be adequately treated in the community because of severe problems which are minimally responsive to intervention. A good deal of neglect of, and lack of concern for, the patients was unearthed. Local programs were seen as not meeting their needs, and an unmet need for hospitalization was noted as well. Hospital closure, the senators concluded, was detrimental to the localities and burdensome to patients, their families, and public officials. Interestingly, they reported that the money saved by closing hospitals was being diverted to programs designed for patients who are easier to manage. One of their major summary statements was: "It is the view of the committee that state hospitals continue to serve as an indispensable component of the mental health system in California."

Wilder[31] has spoken of the necessity for obtaining the advice of the direct consumer in planning for mental health services. It is quite rare for patients to write articles for professional journals, but Allen[32] has done just that. She describes herself as someone who has spent an extended period of time in a California state hospital, and, at the time of writing her paper, was living in a board and care home. It is her position that both hospital and community care are needed and that both need to be improved. She comments about how many patients in board-and-care homes do not take part in the community at all, how these same people may have been active participants in the life of the hospital, and how some show more symptoms which receive less attention. In addition, the author felt more encouragement to express herself freely while in the hospital. Patients will be hurt, we are told, if hospitals don't exist; state hospitals are credited with having a range of facilities that cannot be duplicated by community hospitals.

## New York

In New York, there has also been a marked decline in the census of the state hospitals. Local newspapers frequently carry articles and editorials highly critical of the policies by which patients are returned to communities. But this is not a matter only for the press. The Hospital Committee of the New York County District Branch of the American Psychiatric Association stated that a serious crisis exists in the care of chronic patients, since there are no community-based programs for them.[33] Speaking about children and adolescents, Kalogerakis[34] questions the assumption that seriously disturbed patients can be treated in institutions other than hospitals. He goes on to say that the cutback of inpatient care has already proved injurious.

Another illustration of the lengths of community backlash was provided by the city of Long Beach. An ordinance was passed which was meant to exclude former patients from that city's hotels. A U.S. district court enjoined enforcement of that statute.[35] Documenting the paucity of community agencies equipped to deal with state hospital discharges, Robbins and Robbins[36] tell of the adverse effects on patients, families, and local hospitals. They suggest that the extensive use of the revolving door may be more costly, in a variety of ways, than continuous hospitalization. Reich[37] contends that the burden of care falls to the welfare system, which has no treatment programs available. He concludes: "Our present policy of discharging helpless human beings to a hostile community is immoral and inhumane. It is a return to the Middle Ages, when the mentally ill roamed the streets and little boys threw rocks at them."

Reflecting on a series of meetings held to discuss the problems resulting from efforts to use alternatives to hospitalization and noting signs of increased resistance on the part of localities to receiving discharged patients, McKinley[38] issued the following policy statement for the New York State Department of Mental Hygiene: "Unless we can see a real advantage to the patient in growth toward becoming a more responsible human being, and unless an appropriate and implementable plan to facilitate this growth can be made, we should not take the initiative in discharging the patient to the community." He believes that most of the chronically ill can and should be provided for in communities and recognizes that it is the lack of local resources which causes many patients to return to the hospital.[39]

## Great Britain

I am grateful to Wright[40] for making me aware of the fact that the situation vis-à-vis hospital and community treatment in the United States is paralleled in England. Letemendia and Harris[41] question the applicability of government guidelines for the number of mental hospital beds, demonstrating discrepancies between such figures and actual needs. It is their opinion that the general hospital contribution to reducing the load on the mental hospitals may not turn out to be as large as had been hoped. In a series of letters to the editor following the publication of this paper, Glancy,[42] speaking for the Department of Health and Social Security, attempts to refute some of their statements, but does admit that there are patients who cannot be rehabilitated and for whom prolonged inpatient care will be required; Tredgold[43] points to the need for more community-based staff, without which patients will be returned to hospitals worse off than when they left; Storer[44] indicates that the system is not working well because the services that were to be supplied locally are almost nonexistent; and the original authors[45] make reference to an estimate of the cost of current plans which concludes that, at the present rate of progress, 80 to 100 years may be required as a transitional period. Thus, in Great Britain also, large gaps in service exist, with the development of local programs lagging far behind changes in hospital policy.[46]

Conclusion: At best, the system is not providing well for the severely ill and chronically ill and, at worst, it is a nonsystem.

## Reflections: Past, Present, and Future

Fifteen years ago, Birnbaum[47] proposed the doctrine of the right to treatment, defined as "the legal right of a mentally ill inmate of a public mental institution to adequate medical treatment for his mental illness." The question of whether this right is guaranteed by the Constitution has yet to be addressed by the United States Supreme Court. An increasing number of states, however, are recognizing it by statute.

Two extensions of the concept of the right to treatment have been proposed. Speaking of the patient's right to the right treatment, Bigelow[48] writes: "Just as the generalist does not electively treat malaria in the swamp, nor the dermatologist deal with dermatitis venenata with the patient lying in the poison ivy patch, so the psychiatrist frequently has good reason for removing a patient from a noxious home environment in order to render the right treatment." I have elsewhere[49] recommended: "The concept of the right to adequate treatment . . . must now be extended to include those patients who are involuntarily *communitized*. They do exist, and their needs for comprehensive services are very real, particularly since they are expected to function in the community."

Mayer and Rosenblatt[50] indicate that the history of psychiatric intervention is cyclical. Great claims are made for a new treatment or ideology and, after a period of acceptance and ascendancy, the new approach is questioned. In time, it is overshadowed or replaced, and so it goes. We are at a critical juncture in terms of assessing how well the community mental health movement and the de-emphasis on hospital treatment are meeting the needs of the patients. I submit that much of what is happening today is violative of the right to the right treatment and falls far short of providing adequate treatment to the involuntarily communitized patient.

This review of the literature, although not intended to be exhaustive, is sufficient to demonstrate that for the severely ill and/or chronically recidivistic patient, there are ideological obstacles to hospitalization which may deprive him or her of the type of treatment which may be needed most. Many such patients are in the community in illusion only, where they remain quite symptomatic, and where their presence is not well received by the public, thereby compounding their difficulties. The few treatment programs which are available for such patients often fail in the task of delivering all the necessary services. The questions then become: How did this state of affairs come about? What can be done about it?

Large segments of what can be subsumed under the rubric of the "community mental health movement" are extremely beneficial to those it was designed to serve and represent a tremendous advance over what had been. There are not enough community mental health centers, however, to provide for all of the mental health needs of the country. To discharge patients before treatment programs are available, in the hopes that these programs will develop, or in an attempt to create pressure for services, is to do things backwards. Despite these latter facts, too many of the proponents and advocates of the community approach acted with missionary zeal in promising more than could reasonably be expected and continue to do so while the efficacy of this modality as an alternative to hospitalization for the severely and chronically ill remains unclear.

Widespread dissatisfaction with the level of care in the state hospitals, often in the form of broadside attacks which failed to give due recognition to positive aspects of public mental hospitals, led, in part, to the development of community mental health principles. Perhaps the unhappiness was, more accurately, with our inability to cure, or effectively rehabilitate, many of the hospitalized patients. However, the simple act of discharging patients to the community is, in and of itself, not community psychiatry. The assumption that all patients are better off outside the hospital has been shown to be just that: an assumption. Hospital neglect cannot be replaced by community neglect, and patients should not receive less adequate treatment in the community than they did in the hospital.

Historically, state legislatures have seldom been generous in their appropriations to public mental hospitals, and one result of this policy has been the inability of the hospitals to provide quality care. In these times of governmental financial crisis, it seems politically and economically expedient to advocate the closing of hospitals and the provision of less expensive community care. However, this is tantamount to the abandonment of the needs and rights of those severely and/or chronically ill patients who require hospitalization. If suffering is to be relieved, the quality of life to be improved, and the patient to be helped to take his place in society comfortably, then hospitals must be upgraded. Indeed, for some patients a right to hospitalization might be postulated and, in any event, it is clearly the patient's right to be treated in an environment that is conducive to rapid recovery. Deteriorating physical plants and demoralized staff can hardly be expected to do what is needed. To use the fact that such conditions exist as justification for hospital closure is to attack the effect rather than to remedy the cause.

A community orientation need not, of necessity, include an anti-institutional bias. If it is mental illness that we are attempting to treat, then hospitals are required for some of the patients some of the time. Chronic mental illness will not be eliminated by acts of legislatures, alterations of priorities, shifting of funds, or other bits of prestidigitation. To think otherwise is to do an injustice to the patient as an individual and a disservice to ourselves as professionals.

To set up the equation "community-based *versus* hospital-based" serves only to create a pseudodichotomy. It is patently apparent that both modalities have been, are, and will continue to be essential components of a total service delivery system. The controversy needs to be laid to rest and the rhetoric abandoned.

A full and equal partnership between the state hospital and the community agencies is imperative if any meaningful goals are to be achieved. Each component must be maximally responsive to the needs of the patients both are serving. Inherent in any such proposal is not only the necessity for the patient to be able to move freely back and forth as may be required because of changes in his or her clinical condition, but also equal mobility of staff and money based on demonstrated programmatic requirements rather than on theoretical "white papers." Failing this, all that remains is an untenable alternative: If resources continue to be diverted unidirectionally, we re-create the situation of a two-class system of care whereby the sickest patients are relegated to an underequipped, underfunded, and understaffed public mental hospital, there to be abandoned and forgotten for want of a spokesman.

## References

1. Steinhart, M. J. The selling of community mental health. *Psychiatric Quarterly*, 1973, **47**, 325–340.
2. Black, B. J. Editorial comment: Stop! look! listen! *Psychiatric Quarterly*, 1974, **48**, 295–297.
3. Fischer, A., & Weinstein, M. R. Mental hospitals, prestige, and the image of enlightenment. *Archives of General Psychiatry*, 1971, **25**, 41–48.
4. Bennett, D. Community mental health services in Britain. *American Journal of Psychiatry*, 1973, **130**, 1065–1070.
5. Rachlin, S., Pam, A., & Milton, J. Civil liberties versus involuntary hospitalization. *American Journal of Psychiatry*, 1975, **132**, 189–192.
6. Position statement on involuntary hospitalization of the mentally ill (revised). *American Journal of Psychiatry*, 1973, **130**, 392.
7. Zwerling, I., Karasu, T., Plutchik, R., & Kellerman, S. A comparison of voluntary and involuntary patients in a state hospital. *American Journal of Orthopsychiatry*, 1975, **45**, 81–87.
8. Rosenblatt, A. Providing custodial care for mental patients: An affirmative view. *Psychiatric Quarterly*, 1974, **48**, 14–25.
9. Rosenblatt, A., & Mayer, J. E. The recidivism of mental patients: A review of past studies. *American Journal of Orthopsychiatry*, 1974, **44**, 697–706.
10. Talbott, J. A. Stopping the revolving door—a study of readmissions to a state hospital. *Psychiatric Quarterly*, 1974, **48**, 159–168.
11. Smith, W. G., Kaplan, J., & Siker, D. Community mental health and the seriously disturbed patient. *Archives of General Psychiatry*, 1974, **30**, 693–696.

12. Zwerling, I. Aftercare systems. In S. Arieti (Ed.), *American Handbook of Psychiatry,* (Rev. Ed., Vol. 5). New York: Basic Books, 1975, 721–736.

13. Hogarty, G. E., Goldberg, S. C., Schooler, N. R., Ulrich, R. F., & the Collaborative Study Group. Drug and sociotherapy in the aftercare of schizophrenic patients II. Two year relapse rates. *Archives of General Psychiatry,* 1974, **31,** 603–608.

14. Serban, G., & Thomas, A. Attitudes and behaviors of acute and chronic schizophrenic patients regarding ambulatory treatment. *American Journal of Psychiatry,* 1974, **131,** 991–995.

15. Astrachan, B. M., Brauer, L., Harrow, M., & Schwartz, C. Symptomatic outcome in schizophrenia. *Archives of General Psychiatry,* 1974, **31,** 155–160.

16. Pam, A., Bryskin, L., Rachlin, S., & Rosenblatt, A. Community adjustment of self-discharged patients. *Psychiatric Quarterly,* 1973, **47,** 175–183.

17. Lamb, H. R., & Goertzel, V. Discharged mental patients—are they really in the community? *Archives of General Psychiatry,* 1971, **24,** 29–34.

18. Lamb, H. R., & Goertzel, V. The demise of the state hospital—a premature obituary? *Archives of General Psychiatry,* 1972, **26,** 489–495.

19. Rabkin, J. Public attitudes toward mental illness: A review of the literature. *Schizophrenia Bulletin,* Fall 1974, issue **10,** 9–33.

20. Bentz, W. K., & Edgerton, J. W. Consensus on attitudes toward mental illness. *Archives of General Psychiatry,* 1970, **22,** 468–473.

21. Mosher, L. R., & Gunderson, J. G. Special report: Schizophrenia, 1972. *Schizophrenia Bulletin,* Winter 1973, issue **7,** 12–52.

22. The relatives of schizophrenics. *Lancet,* 1974, **II,** 33.

23. Kreisman, D. E., & Joy, V. D. Family response to the mental illness of a relative: A review of the literature. *Schizophrenia Bulletin,* Fall 1974, issue **10,** 34–57.

24. Rabiner, C. J., & Lurie, A. The case for psychiatric hospitalization. *American Journal of Psychiatry,* 1974, **131,** 761–764.

25. Modlin, H. C. Balancing patients' rights with the rights of others. *Hospital and Community Psychiatry,* 1974, **25,** 474–475.

26. Rachlin, S. On the need for a closed ward in an open hospital: The psychiatric intensive care unit. *Hospital and Community Psychiatry,* 1973, **24,** 829–833.

27. Birnbaum, M. The right to treatment: Some comments on its development. In F. J. Ayd (Ed.), *Medical, Moral and Legal Issues in Mental Health Care.* Baltimore: Williams and Wilkins, 1974, 97–141.

28. Aviram, U., & Segal, S. P. Exclusion of the mentally ill. *Archives of General Psychiatry,* 1973, **29,** 126–131.

29. Abramson, M. F. The criminalization of mentally disordered behavior: Possible side-effect of a new mental health law. *Hospital and Community Psychiatry,* 1972, **23,** 101–105.

30. Final report to the California legislature of the Senate Select Committee on Proposed Phaseout of State Hospital Services. Sacramento, California, March 15, 1974.

31. Wilder, J. F. *Consumer evaluation of mental health services.* Presented as the Fifteenth Annual Bertram H. Roberts Memorial Lecture, Department of Psychiatry, Yale University, New Haven, Connecticut, May 1971.

32. Allen, P. A consumer's view of California's mental health care system. *Psychiatric Quarterly,* 1974, **48,** 1–13.

33. New York psychiatrists criticize phase-out of state hospital beds (news and notes). *Hospital and Community Psychiatry,* 1973, **24,** 56–60.

34. Kalogerakis, M. G. Still needed for New York: A new deal for the severely disturbed child. *Bulletin of New York State District Branches, American Psychiatric Association,* 1974, **17** (4), 4–6.

35. City restrained from barring mental patients. *Psychiatric News,* July 3, 1974, 1.
36. Robbins, E., & Robbins, L. Charge to the community: Some early effects of a state hospital system's change of policy. *American Journal of Psychiatry,* 1974, **131**, 641–645.
37. Reich, R. Care of the chronically mentally ill—a national disgrace. *American Journal of Psychiatry,* 1973, **130**, 911–912.
38. McKinley, R. A. Memorandum to hospital directors. Albany, State of New York, Department of Mental Hygiene, February 22, 1974.
39. McKinley, R. A. Written communication. October 24, 1974.
40. Wright, J. B. Written communication. November 1, 1974.
41. Letemendia, F. J. J., & Harris, A. D. Psychiatric services and the future. *Lancet,* 1973, **II**, 1013–1016.
42. Glancy, J. E. McA. Psychiatric services and the future (letter to ed.). *Lancet,* 1974, **I**, 510.
43. Tredgold, R. F. Psychiatric services and the future (letter to ed.). *Lancet,* 1974, **I**, 801–802.
44. Storer, D. Psychiatric services and the future (letter to ed.). *Lancet,* 1974, **I**, 802.
45. Letemendia, F. J. J., & Harris, A. D. Psychiatric services and the future (letter to ed.). *Lancet,* 1974, **I**, 1227–1228.
46. Mental hospitals and community services (notes and news). *Lancet,* 1974, **I**, 1124.
47. Birnbaum, M. The right to treatment. *American Bar Association Journal,* 1960, **46**, 499–505.
48. Bigelow, N. Editorial comment: The right to the right treatment. *Psychiatric Quarterly,* 1970, **44**, 533–549.
49. Rachlin, S. With liberty and psychosis for all. *Psychiatric Quarterly,* 1974, **48**, 410–420.
50. Mayer, J. E., & Rosenblatt, A. Clash in perspective between mental patients and staff. *American Journal of Orthopsychiatry,* 1974, **44**, 432–441.

# 5

# The Alternative Care Is Not There

PAUL R. DINGMAN

Although historical developments are covered in some detail in another chapter, it may be useful to re-emphasize that state mental hospitals were, at their inception, highly successful. That success was not due either to an "illness" conception of psychological disorder nor to a "moral therapy" conception of its remediation, but to the great compassion of those physicians of the time who agreed to care for the mentally disordered. They provided the psychologically crippled with a kindly, consistent, and somewhat sheltered, but essentially ordinary living situation. Today, most of us would call this "providing an environment in which growth can occur" rather than "moral therapy."[1]

No matter, results in the early years were excellent. Studies in the first decade at Worcester State Hospital, for example, showed recovery rates in excess of 50%. Independent follow-up studies of Worcester State Hospital patrons made some decades later yielded similar results.[2]

With a rapidly expanding total population, and with the initial successes, the state hospitals were soon overwhelmed by demands for admission. The subsequent overcrowding and the decline in appropriations relative to the size of institution populations made it impossible to continue the kind of benign and consistent surroundings which had

PAUL R. DINGMAN • University Counseling Center, Colgate University, Hamilton, New York 13346.

been the basis of the initial success. Decline in the quality of care provided was immediately evident. Perhaps the whole plan of care by state hospitals should have been abandoned at that time along with the existing facilities.

But it was not. Despite its obvious weaknesses, the plan expanded rapidly and continued to expand for over 100 years. In that period, there were many undesirable developments. There were also, however, significant desirable developments, and a great deal of useful and commendable service was rendered (to be outlined in a later section). By 1955, some 500,000 Americans were being served in state mental hospitals at any one time.

Then suddenly the trend reversed and the daily censuses began to drop. Today the total daily census in state mental institutions is probably under 220,000.

It is popular to attribute this new trend to the wholesale introduction of psychotropic drugs. Whether it is related, either directly or indirectly, remains open to question. Morton Kramer[3] points out that the trend had already begun before the significant and extensive use of the drugs had taken place. Lawrence Kubie[4] points out the difficulties in assessing the apparent value of drugs. Certainly the number of studies which meet his criteria for careful research is not large.

A number of factors may have served to improve treatment and therefore to have increased discharge rates. One of these was the booming economy of the United States during the decade following World War II. Some states were able to increase the operating budgets of their hospital systems by 200% and more.

Another factor was the reaping of the harvest of federally sponsored higher education. Before the World War II, for example, qualified clinical psychologists numbered, at most, in the hundreds. By 1955, they numbered in the thousands. Over 1,200 had been qualified by the American Board, established in the late 1940s. Similar increases, perhaps even more dramatic, could be found in other psychoprofessional fields.

Still another factor was the advent of the 8-hour day and 40-hour week in state institutions, which brought major changes in atmosphere and attitudes. Unfortunately, it also virtually doubled unit costs.

Rising costs more than any other factor have finally made it obvious that support of state mental hospitals is politically unfeasible. (Only for a brief period at the time of their inception was their support politically popular). This appears to be the principal factor behind the present push to get rid of the state hospitals.

But why are psychoprofessionals so enthusiastic about closing the state hospitals? Are they actually so responsive to political realities?

Probably not. Probably the clamor to get on the "close-the-state-hospital" bandwagon is simply another expression of the glee with which psychoprofessionals seek out new fads, as they did with electroshock, insulin, lobotomy, orgone therapy, "touchy-feely" groups, and what have you.

The legitimate and necessary functions evolved by the state hospitals can be outlined briefly. Those on which there is pretty common agreement are as follows:

1. *Respite.* Although there is a great deal of discussion about the effect of family and local environment on psychological well-being, relatively little attention is given to the use of the hospital as a haven from pressures for temporary periods. Experience has demonstrated repeatedly that brief freedom from pressures can make possible the reorganization of one's strengths so that he can cope fruitfully. In this way, extensive psychological crippling can often be avoided. Fortunately, we are beginning again to get research bearing on this aspect of hospital care. In this connection the work of Lowell Cooper[5] is of interest, showing significant changes during brief hospitalization.

2. *Treatment.* The advantages and disadvantages of hospitalization during the course of treatment need not be reviewed here. Simply the reminder needs to be offered that there are numerous situations in which hospitalization is advantageous, and others in which it is necessary in order for treatment to proceed. Among these would be the case of psychotherapy during periods of distraught and unpredictable behavior. Without hospitalization, psychotherapy must either be temporarily delayed or operate with handicap. Another example is in drug use where 24-hour monitoring of physiological and psychological response to various drugs and dosages may be required. (The foregoing is not in any sense a justification for *commitment,* which will be discussed later.)

3. *Protection of the individual.* The need of some people for protection at various times in their lives from undue pressure by relatives, or from being taken advantage of by others in business or personal relationships, is clear enough. It is all very well to plan to change families and societies so that these people will always be treated fairly and kindly. Until our plans have begun to bear demonstrable fruit, however, it is necessary to continue to provide for them the less than optimal protection of the state mental hospital.

4. *Protection of others.* The necessity for society to be protected from officially recognized and classified psychotics has, of course, been grossly overdrawn. That fact, however, does not make the necessity disappear altogether. Unless we are able to establish satisfactory jail facilities or to devise other means of control and supervision for the few

cases, it will continue to be necessary to provide for detaining them in state hospitals. Failure to attend to this necessity increases public misunderstanding. It appears to have been a major factor in Governor Reagan's recent decision to halt plans to phase out California's mental hospitals.[7]

5. *Research.* The necessity to have numbers of varied subjects available on a continuous basis for research to be undertaken does not require detailed discussion here. Nor does the record of mental hospital staffs in generating the bulk of the research on human personality and human psychological miseries require defending.

6. *Technical training.* Virtually all of us owe most, if not all, of our training experience to facilities which were state mental hospitals or which shared state mental hospital characteristics in essentials. Certain aspects of what we learned simply would not have been learned without close contact for long periods with a variety of chronically disturbed individuals.

7. *Long-term care for chronically disturbed individuals.* In discussing this problem recently at a conference on the future roles of state hospitals held at Buffalo, Cumming[8] indicated that this care must be provided by "the same people who take care of the acutely mentally ill." He was speaking to the point that we cannot with logic expect others to take much interest in those in whom we refuse to take interest.

Even if the limitations, the shortcomings, and the abuses of state hospitals are taken as sufficient cause for decision to abandon this mode of service, there are ethical and moral considerations which dictate against shutting them down on any major scale. In supporting the existence and the utilization of state hospitals, many kinds of commitments, both expressed and implied, have been made.

To begin with, workers on many levels and in many fields have been encouraged to prepare themselves in specific kinds of work in specific settings. Therefore, when a hospital closes, it is not enough to say that these workers will be placed in "similar" jobs in other settings. Nor is it enough to say that the department will "make sure they are not hurt economically." Even in the case in which a worker gets a job with the same job title and the same seniority on paper, he cannot be said to have the same position he formerly had. There is a substantial literature on the economic and psychological consequences of being uprooted from one's work which cannot be ignored. Additionally, self-interest demands recognition that the enthusiasm with which workers join us in our future endeavors will be related to the manner in which we deal with our commitments to present workers.

Further, the impact of a hospital's closing must inevitably have profound impact on the surrounding community. Dozens of towns in the United States owe their existence entirely or principally to a state hospital. Virtually everyone serves the hospital as a worker, or indirectly, as a supplier of goods or services. In dozens of other localities, the state hospital has provided the largest single source of demand for the development of supply systems, educational systems, and so on. The ecological impact of a state hospital closing is unassessable, staggering, incredible in its proportions. The fact that state departments have no notion as to how to meet our obligation to these communities does not make the obligation go away.

Finally, the most critical ethical consideration for the professional when a hospital is to be closed must be the well-being of his individual patrons. None would hold that an action, such as closing an institution, could be justified ethically on the basis that it would be best for a majority, or best in the long run, if the immediate effect were harmful to the individual patron. Other chapters provide information on the well-being of patrons who have been put out of state hospitals because of closings. They do not, however, describe in detail the filthy conditions in fourth-rate hotels used for scores, or hundreds, of former mental hospital patients.[9] Nor do they describe the dungeonlike basement conditions in which some are surviving in unlicensed, semirural "permit" homes in many states.

Two kinds of illustrations point up the lack of likelihood for appropriate new arrangements for those now served by hospitals. First let us look at the recommendations of professionals as to the proper management for patients at present being served by a mental hospital. For that purpose the tabulation of patients of St. Elizabeth's hospital prepared in 1973 by Taube and Pollack[10] will serve.

The recommended placement categories were:

| | |
|---|---|
| Own home or apartment, etc. | 12.6% |
| Foster home | 34.6 |
| Nursing homes | 20.7 |
| Psychiatric hospital | 32.1 |

Can these people actually be placed as recommended? Many optimists would agree that 13% of the residents of our typical hospitals could be placed essentially on their own. However, few would be optimistic about locating foster homes for 35% of all their patrons.

Experience has shown that nursing homes are generally already full to capacity. Furthermore, nursing homes do not want people who have

been identified as mental hospital patients. They are accepted only
reluctantly, under pressure, and only with promises of consultation and
the option of returning the person to the state's care.

And what about the remaining third who are seen as continuing to
require hospitalization? Is it realistic to assume that they can be transferred to other state hospitals or to local mental hospital facilities? Is it
not the case that all are now overcrowded and understaffed?

It is clearly not realistic to assume that most present mental hospital
patrons can be placed in appropriate recommended placements. Therefore, when a hospital is closed, inappropriate placements will be inevitable.

The second illustration is a concrete case from recent experience.
When Grafton State Hospital began the process of phasing out its entire
operation in the spring of 1971, it was operating two special residences
on its grounds. These residences were in many ways similar to the
"quarter-way" house program described in *Social Work* by Michael
Wiernasz.[11] There were however some unusual features in these two
residences. The patients were free to select their own physicians from
the medical staff and they had a choice of independent food preparation, participation in a communal kitchen, or access to the institution
cafeteria. Patrons of these two residences were "temporarily" transferred to the wards of another state hospital, pending the establishing
of additional halfway facilities in the community (Grafton had only one
in operation at the time). Some 24 months later, all were still living on
the wards with no prospects in sight for the promised halfway houses.

The reasons for difficulties in acquiring sites for halfway houses
will have to be examined later. It is intended here to illustrate only that
patrons are going to be hurt when institutions are closed, even with
careful planning and the best of intentions.

The case for state mental hospitals must include study of the
reasons why they have poorly, often abysmally, carried out the functions outlined above. Since hope for successful transfer of functions has
been raised, it will be important to learn, also, whether the defects and
weaknesses we find in the mental hospitals exist in other organizations
as well. Particularly we will be concerned with the comprehensive
community mental health center. This new darling of the psychoestab-
lishment is the most popular nominee to carry on the functions to be
abandoned by state mental hospitals. Point-by-point comparison
reveals that the problems of the state hospitals have already begun to
show themselves in the CCMHCs.

1. It has been pointed out that ownership and form of organization
disposes the state mental hospital toward poor work. Being monolithic

and authoritarian, it is sensitive only to the pressures of bureaucracy and politics and, hence, is rigid and inflexible. Unfortunately, guidelines for the distribution of federal funds made the control of CCMHCs by university medical schools and by private general hospitals inevitable. Both of these are, in their own right, excellent examples of monolithic and authoritarian structures. Hence the situation has arisen in which Perlmutter and Silverman[12] aptly describes the CCMHC as a "structural anachronism" that hinders research and limits responsiveness to changing environmental conditions. It is, in effect, an agent to promote the status quo, they say. Stefanos[13] describes in detail the impossibility for a citizen's corporation to become a CCMHC. He believes the "so-called CCMHC is doomed to failure . . . [precisely] because it was *not* developed by its community." Vaughan[14] describes the ultimate perversion in which a CCMHC is totally owned and operated by a corporation of psychiatrists in private practice. (His is by no means the only illustration of that occurrence.)

2. State hospitals have been criticized as being poorly located and having outdated facilities. These would not appear to be central criticisms. They are simply indications of the unwillingness of legislative bodies to appropriate funds necessary for relocation and updating of facilities. Insofar as inappropriate methods are perpetuated by inappropriate physical facilities, the CCMHC is already in serious trouble. More important, it shares the crippling defect of low political popularity. Some citizens were misled by Washington rhetoric of the earlier 1960s and thought that federal funding would both stimulate and partially replace local and state funding. Federal appropriations for CCMHC construction and staffing were never high enough to sustain widespread change, however. The fleeting interest of politicians has pretty much vanished, and there is no particular reason to expect it to return (see discussions below of costs and of unworkable principles shared by both institutions). For example, according to Demone and Schulberg[15] the legislature of the progressive state of Massachusetts is designating 80% of all Department of Mental Health funds specifically for state mental hospitals.

3. The state mental hospital has been criticized in that its operation has apparently encouraged disproportionate rates of commitment whereby the poor become vastly overrepresented in the hospital population. There is no question that the phenomenon exists, but it is not a mental hospital phenomenon as such. Lorion has shown, in his review of the literature of the past decade,[16] that the mode of treatment in community facilities is strongly influenced by socioeconomic status. Sheely and Wright[17] demonstrated in Georgia that community facilities

are proportionately more readily available to persons considered "white." This probably influences referral and commitment to mental hospitals which are disproportionately heavily populated by "blacks."

4. It is easy to show that state mental hospitals, being geographically distant (from the most heavily populated areas), are not readily accessible to most people to assist in the management of psychological emergencies. No one would deny that. But the implication that CCMHCs are readily available for psychological emergencies is simply not warranted. Gerald Jacobson indicates in a recent issue of the *American Journal of Public Health*[18] that the emergency services of CCMHCs are poorly defined and carried out without enthusiasm, if at all, although these services are understood to be a required part of the activity of federally funded CCMHCs. Jacobson quotes Glasscote in pointing out that six of eight centers surveyed "provided" emergency services in a general hospital emergency room without the actual presence there of mental hospital personnel. None of the eight had mental health professionals available around the clock. Jacobson believes that the very poor record of service of the CCMHCs in this area is attributable in large measure to the low regard in which such service is held by psychoprofessionals and to the resulting assignment to the emergency services of the lowest status staff.

5. The state mental hospital is criticized for its failure to provide "continuity of care." By this is meant that (a) it is unusual for a state hospital to admit a person immediately upon the recommendation alone of a worker not on its own staff, and (b) it is extremely difficult for a state hospital staff to obtain the assistance of local organizations in serving people who leave the state hospital.

For the latter reason, many state hospitals have established systems of "aftercare" both on their own grounds and in the local areas which they serve. Many of these aftercare services do very poor work. Some do excellent work.

The proponents of CCMHCs would have us believe that the patrons of these organizations can simply and easily have access to office visit service, hospital care, day hospital care, family social service help, and a variety of other kinds of special services. Further, they would have us believe that the work of each is neatly related, even subordinated if necessary, to the other. In fact, of course, the staffs of the individual services can be just as possessive of their patrons and just as uncooperative with each other as they are with the staffs of state mental hospitals.

It is difficult to separate fact from slogan in this area. Bass and

Windle[19] have attempted to work out a quantitative measure of care continuity. I read their discussion of the necessity to promote continuity as indicating some reservation about the actual existence of this phenomenon.

A strong case can be made for the view that neither the form of organization nor the mechanisms of transfer have anything to do with continuity of care. From the patron's point of view, continuity of care would probably mean having a professional whom he could depend upon to continue to serve him, regardless of which of the facilities he happened to be using at any given time. Professional workers who are willing to render such service probably are quite rare. Even if they could be located, the managements of the various service components would very thoroughly discourage them. Management finds great difficulty in paying salaries to workers for service to people who are statistics on some other organization's books, especially if the work is carried out on the other organization's turf.

6. Related to the continuity problem are the problems of access and choice. The ethical statements of the American Psychological Association, the American Medical Association, the American Bar Association, and probably other groups require that a person have free access to and free choice of professionals to serve him. Mental hospitals routinely reject these requirements (if a person is committed, he is not even permitted to refuse to see the professional who is assigned to him). The effectiveness of the work, of course, suffers from this. The CCMHC treats people essentially in the same manner. Those which are not monolithic form themselves into cartellike consortiums. These treat the individual essentially as the baseball cartel treats the player. In our case, however, the "yellow-dog contract," with its "reserve clause," is seldom put on paper. Instead, the patron is told, indirectly, that if he does not like the selection of professionals made for him, he may decline to be served by that professional. If he does so, however, no staff member of any group within the cartel will ever see him either.

7. The state mental hospital has been justly criticized because of its poor record of demonstrable results. Just how the CCMHC compares is difficult to assess because the populations differ so greatly. One might choose to believe that the populations differ because the state mental hospitals like to gobble up the poor and the helpless. Or he could believe that it is also partly because community services tend to push such people away from them. The statistical observations of Sheely and Wright[20] would tend to support the latter rather than the former. In studies in which the same individuals are observed over a long period,

as in the work of Davis, Dinitz, and Pasamanick,[21] differences in the social or psychological functioning of those served in a community-based program and those served in a mental hospital cannot be found. This ought not to be surprising since Barrett, Kuriansky, and Gurland show quite clearly that survival in the community is related to the function the individual has in the family with which he lives.[22] This is unlikely to be differentially influenced by hospital and community-based services.

8. One hears talk that state hospitals are "too expensive" and that CCMHCs can "do the job" at lower cost. Of course, it is difficult to pin down that kind of talk. On the other hand, state hospitals cost too little, so little ($4,000 to $18,000 per patient-year) that it is patently impossible to carry out high-quality, intensive work. On the other hand, because clear-cut comparison studies are impossible to achieve, the most rational assumption is that identical work under one kind of management would cost about the same as under another. Kubie has expressed that view with some vehemence.[23] Alexander and Sheely demonstrate it with some precision regarding a variety of services as rendered in private practice and by a CCMHC.[24]

9. Size has always been a problem for state hospitals. Initially, they underestimated the scope of the problem, thinking that one, or at the most two or three, facilities could serve an entire state. Being without the means of limiting admissions within those areas, they found that their populations quickly grew so large as to preclude reasonable service.[25] CCMHCs have dealt with part of the problem by limiting, in their charters, the total population to be served. It is hoped that their estimates will prove more durable than those of the state hospitals.

More important than gross numbers of cases are the quality of staff and the ratio of workers to patrons. The inadequacies of state hospitals in these respects, of course, led directly to various abuses: inadequacy or absence of treatment, cynicism and lack of concern on the part of the staff, dehumanizing environments, failure to protect patrons against brutality, and others.

Although it is by no means exhaustive, the foregoing material illustrates that the defects of state mental hospitals are likely to be transferred along with their functions to CCMHCs. In summary, one might ask the following questions: Would it not have been possible for anyone familiar with mental hospital work to have predicted with some precision the gullibility and rigidity of staff members described in Rosenhan's account of the experiences of eight subjects who gained admission to hospitals under false pretenses by complaining of hearing voices?[26] Would anyone active in CCMHC work be surprised if Rosenhan were able to obtain from a similar study of CCMHCs essentially the same results? Is there anything about them which would make them less vulnerable?

Finally, we need to be aware of three sets of misconceptions or trends of thinking which underlie the problems indicated and which have made it impossible for state mental hospitals to be more effective in reducing misery and promoting well-being.

The first of these is that mental disorders are illnesses—"just like any other illness." State institutions were early committed to this conception, and cemented it with the "hospital" designation and the use of physicians as superintendents. These physicians of the early 19th century held all illnesses, including psychological distress, to be due to failure to live in strict accord with natural laws ordained by God. Hence, treatment of all disorders required that the "patients" be guided in living proper, ordered lives—as understood by these religious men. That was the essence of "moral therapy."

As the moral conception of pathology in general gave way to mechanical, chemical, and physiological conceptions of pathology, mental troubles were carried along. The results were that, to this day, psychoprofessionals have been trying to force psychological miseries into often inappropriate classification schemes and have been tagging people with labels based on these schemes. The labels influence not at all the mode of treatment selected. Because the labeling system is irrational, however, it is quite difficult to remove the labels once applied (it requires courage to aver that someone is *no longer* "schizophrenic," even subclinically, if he has ever been so labeled, or *no longer* "depressed").

More important, the continuation of the "illness" notion has resulted in the perpetuation of hope for simple mechanical, chemical, or physiological "cures" for psychological troubles. It has kept the energy and attention of mental hospitals from the study of social and psychological forces and from the application of already existing knowledge.

Szasz[27] and Albee[28] have outlined the fallacies inherent in the notion of "mental illness," and the impossibility of generating effective means of helping from this conceptual base. I do not wish to add more here except to call attention to a recent discussion by Waitzkin[29] which shows from a somewhat different point of view how the existence of a "sickness" role serves to keep a person from making progress, rather than to bring about change in him.

Perhaps a factor tending to hold the "mental illness" notion in place is the belief that the general public can tolerate an "illness" conception more readily than it can tolerate a "psychological disorder" conception. Actually, ordinary people were never much fooled by the "illness" label. They simply substituted the word *sick* for the words *crazy* or *loony* when in the company of psychoprofessionals or other sophisticates and continued to think of these conditions in the same terms they always had.

To the extent that community services hold to this conception, their work must suffer as has that of the mental hospitals. The pressure for CCMHCs to go along is very great. Most are budgeted on the premise that there will be considerable income from insurance, prepayment plans, and other third parties. All of these require that the center certify that the person being served has an "illness." Even if the center itself could decide to forgo this income, associated groups would be insistent. United Campaigns and United Givers' Funds, for example, typically insist on helping out only on a "deficit budgeting" basis. This means their share of the funding will be forthcoming only after all other possible sources, legitimate or otherwise, have been demonstrated to be exhausted. School systems press the center for absence excuses based on "illness." They hope thereby to avoid invoking truant regulations and court problems, questioning from bureaucrats further up in the hierarchy, and the potential loss of state reimbursement funds. And, so far, the centers have had essentially no outside help in resisting. The outlook is not hopeful.

Second, the acceptance of involuntary confinement has diminished the effectiveness of the state hospital. Edwalds has written that the primary social functions of a state mental hospital are not necessarily the officially stated purposes and goals.[30] The primary functions are defined by the nature of the authority and the power delegated to the institution by society—in other words, what society demands. The secondary functions of the institution constitute whatever services the institution is able to render with the facilities that happen to be available.

Edwalds defines the primary functions of state hospitals as: (1) public safety and the removal from society of individuals showing certain kinds of disruptive behavior, and (2) custodial care. Edwalds believes that there has been no change in these primary social demands in the past 100 years. He calls treatment and rehabilitation "at best, secondary social functions." The institution, however, officially believes them to be primary. In the resulting self-deception and confusion, high-quality management and treatment are not possible. I would go further and say that commitment virtually excludes the possibility of treatment. If an institution accepts custody or commitment of a person, a relationship is established which shares characteristics of a family relationship.

It is the familylike relationship which precludes treatment, since one may not serve professionally the members of his own family. A long history of human tragedy has led to the inclusion of this principle in the ethical standards of most professions.

Very few discussions dealing with the dilemma of trying to serve both parental and therapeutic functions are available. Some suggestions for practical exploration are offered by Zober and Tabor.[31]

Laws governing commitment are now undergoing changes in many states. The changes are a good sign, but the fact of involuntary confinement supported by law remains. If state hospitals are discontinued, there will be great pressure on community services to accept commitments of one kind or another.

Will the kindly CCMHC directors of tomorrow be able to resist what kindly state hospital superintendents could not resist 150 years ago? Or will they accept the "primary functions" left behind by the state hospital?

The third concern centers around usurpation of the right to help.[32] A logical analysis would award the right to help in a sequence something like this: first to the individual who has the problem, next to his family and close friends, next to his neighbors and other natural groups such as co-workers, and finally to society as represented by political entities.

Where does the person with special technical skills, the professional, fit in? Logically, the professional belongs only where he is asked to serve by the one who has the right to help.[33] Historically, things have worked out differently. We seem always to have had with us those with a "calling" or a "profession" who consider themselves more deeply concerned with helping than is the ordinary person. Professionals feel that their charitable impulses are not only stronger, but of an entirely different, and higher, quality than those of the lay person. (Let us be charitable and comment only that they have confused a technical skill with a virtue.) Accordingly, they have been impelled, when a problem appears and an ordinary citizen is trying to help, to step in and take over.

It is but a short step, then, to an arrogant possessiveness expressed in terms such as "my client," "my case," or "my patient," and from there to the view that the problem and its management are the property of the worker, not of the customer. As professionals have gained more and more control, the individual with the problem is in deeper and deeper trouble.

Examples can be found in several fields of virtually complete control being exercised over the individual in the name of "helping." Fischer describes conceptual and functional similarities between men-

tal institutions and public schools—both of which have captive customers.[34] He points to control by superiors, pressure for conformity,
labeling, drugging, isolation, and surveillance and record-keeping as
actions which are justified as helpful to the customer but which are
typically dehumanizing. In reality they are done to make life easier for
the professional.

Mayhon and others describe how professional social service workers rob citizens of the privilege, the pleasure, and the responsibility of
helping neighbors in distress, thereby preventing the development of
their abilities and creating dependence on the professionals.[35] Fortunately, the same work also describes processes by which the right to
help can be given back to its original owners. The authors show that it
is possible thereby to develop new and equally gratifying work for the
professionals.

Mental hospital professionals are classic in their arrogations. They
fight among themselves over who shall control the patron. They make
treaties ceding certain property rights to each other. They join forces to
deny beachheads to third groups. They even form multiprofessional
alliances designed to still any voice of protest from the most peripheral
groups. In emergencies, staff members are assigned to organize "citizen participation" programs. These appoint the more persistent and
vocal citizens to "lay advisory councils" (with predictable results), and
arrange for the others to serve as "lay volunteers" who will work in
canteens, read to old folks, etc.

The taint of this professional arrogance has followed psychoprofessionals as they have moved out from hospital work into community
settings. It tends to be reinforced by associates in general hospitals,
social services, schools, and so on. If the trend cannot be reversed, the
effectiveness of the psychoprofessionals in community settings can
never rise above that achieved by them in mental hospital settings.

The psychoprofessional must accept as his ultimate goal to make it
easier for others to carry out their own charitable impulses, and to help
each to find the best way to relieve the suffering of his neighbors. In
whatever capacity the citizen chooses to become involved, the job of the
professional is to assist in the creation of an environment in which both
paid and unpaid workers may assist individuals to develop to their
fullest. He must be willing to give up the pleasure of assisting directly,
because the citizen has more right to that pleasure than the professional. In turn, he can expect to find new satisfactions, one of which is
assisting citizens to assume responsibility, to progress, and to grow.

It is hoped that this outline, together with the other presentations
in this volume, will help to strengthen the resolve not to waste energy

in the futile exercise of "closing the state mental hospitals," but rather to renew efforts to develop effective means of reducing psychological misery to the end, in part, that those institutions may simply pass away as their patrons leave and their services are no longer sought by anyone. Interesting new service plans based on new conceptions—some of which are already developed to the stage of sophisticated trial applications—*are* offered frequently in our journals. We *can* move forward, and we can simultaneously honor past commitments, however foolishly made.

To recapitulate:

1. State mental hospitals *do* exist, we have encouraged dependence upon them, and they do perform necessary and legitimate functions.
2. Suitable alternative facilities do not exist at this time.
3. CCMHCs are inheriting many of the defects of state mental hospitals. There is little point in planning to transfer functions to them, unless the defects can be remedied.
4. Closings on any major scale are unthinkable.
5. There are leads that are still free from the crippling thinking of the past which we can explore. We have every reason to hope that we can build new and more effective means of relieving psychological misery.

## References

1a. Betts, C., & Dingman, P. R. The nursing role in a children's day hospital. *Journal of Psychiatric Nursing*, 1969, **7**, 22–24.

1b. Cumming, J. Milieu therapy in the hospital and the community. In J. Zusman (Chairman), *The state hospital—past and present*. Willard State Hospital Centennial Symposium, Sandoz, Hanover, New Jersey, 1974.

1c. Dingman, P. . Environmental requirements for psychological growth. *Journal of Clinical Child Psychology*, 1971, **1**, 3–4.

2. Grob, G. N. *Mental institutions in America: Social policy to 1875*. New York: Free Press, 1973.

3. Kramer, M., & Pollack, E. S. Problems in the interpretation of trends in the population movement of the public mental hospitals. *American Journal of Public Health*, 1958, **48**(8), 1003–1019.

4. Kubie, L. Pitfalls of community psychiatry. *Archives of General Psychiatry*, 1969, **18**, 257–265.

5. Cooper, L. Cognitive changes during acute psychiatric hospitalization. *Journal of Clinical Psychology*, 1973, **29**(1), 26–27.

6. Graham, J. R., Lilly, R. S., Konick, D. S., Paolino, A. F., & Friedman, I. M.M.P.I. changes associated with short-term psychiatric hospitalization. *Journal of Clinical Psychology* 1973, **29**(1), 69–73.

7. Reagan reneges. *American Psychological Association Monitor*, 1974, **4**, 1, 7.

8. Cumming, J. Who will care for the chronically mentally ill? In J. Zusman (Ed.), *The future role of the state hospital.* Buffalo: State University of New York at Buffalo, 1973.
9. Zusman, J. (Chairman). Introduction. In *The state hospital—past and present.* Willard State Hospital Centennial Symposium, Sandoz, Hanover, New Jersey, 1974.
10. Taube, C. A., & Pollack, E. S. Trends and projections in state hospital use. In J. Zusman (Ed.), *The future role of the state hospital.* Buffalo: State University at Buffalo, 1973.
11. Wiernasz, M. J. Quarterway-house program for the hospitalized mentally ill. *Social Work,* 1972, **17**(6), 72–77.
12. Perlmutter, F., & Silverman, H. A. C.MH.C.: A structural anachronism. *Social Work,* 1972, **17**(2), 78–84.
13. Stephanos, R. C. Citizens' corporations as true community mental retardation and mental health centers. *Mental Hygiene,* 1971, **55**(3), 410–412.
14. Vaughan, W. T., Newman, D. C., Levy, A., & Marty, S. Private practice of community psychiatry. *American Journal of Psychiatry,* 1973, **130**(1), 24–27.
15. Demone, H. W., & Schulberg, H. D. Massachusetts' ten year human services plan. In J. Zusman (Ed.), *The future role of the state hospital.* Buffalo: State University at Buffalo, 1973.
16. Lorion, R. P. Socioeconomic status and traditional treatment approaches reconsidered. *Psychological Bulletin,* 1973, **79**(4), 263–270.
17. Sheely, A., & Wright, P. A. State-wide epidemiological assessment of the effectiveness of community mental health services. *Journal of Clinical Psychology,* 1972, **18** (1), 109–111.
18. Jacobson, G. F. Emergency services in community mental health. *American Journal of Public Health,* 1974, **64**(2), 124–128.
19. Bass, R. D., & Windle, C. A. Preliminary attempt to measure continuity of care in a community mental health center. *Community Mental Health Journal,* 1973, **9**(1), 53–62.
20. Sheely, A., & Wright, P. A. State-wide epidemiological assessment of the effectiveness of community mental health services. *Journal of Clinical Psychology,* 1972, **28** (1), 109–111.
21. Davis, A. E., Dinitz, S., & Pasamanick, E. The prevention of hospitalization in schizophrenia: Five years after an experimental program. *American Journal of Orthopsychiatry,* 1972, **42**(3), 375–388.
22. Barrett, J. E., Kuriansky, J., & Gurland, B. Community tenure following emergency discharge. *American Journal of Psychiatry,* 1972, **128**(8), 958–964.
23. Kubie, L. Pitfalls of community psychiatry. *Archives of General Psychiatry,* 1969, **18**, 257–265.
24. Alexander, R. J., & Sheely, M. D. Cost per hour for delivery of service in a community mental health center. *Diseases of the Nervous System,* 1971, **32**(11), 769–776.
25a. Grob, G. N. *Mental institutions in America: Social policy to 1875.* New York: Free Press, 1973.
25b. Grob, G. N. *Worcester State Hospital in Massachusetts, 1830–1920.* Chapel Hill: University of North Carolina Press, 1966.
26a. Rosenhan, D. L. One being sane in insane places. *Science.* 1973, **179**(4070), 250–258.
26b. Sheely, A., & Wright, P. A. State-wide epidemiological assessment of the effectiveness of community mental health services. *Journal of Clinical Psychology,* 1972, **28** (1), 109–111.
27. Szasz, R. S. *The myth of mental illness.* New York: Paul B. Hoeber, Harper and Brothers, 1961.

28. Albee, G. W. Emerging concepts of mental illness and models of treatment: The psychological point of view. *American Journal of Psychiatry,* 1969, **125**(7), 870–875.
29. Waitzkin, H. Latent function of the sick role in various institutional settings. *Social Science and Medicine,* 1971, **5**(1), 45–75.
30. Edwalds, R. M. Functions of the state mental hospital as a social institution. *Mental Hygiene,* 1964, **48,** 666–671.
31. Zober, E., & Tabor, M. The child welfare agency as parent. *Child Welfare,* 1965, **44,** 387–391.
32. Dingman, P. R., Mayhon, J., & Soules, S. *Who has the right to help? Principles involved in volunteer programs.* Discussion presented at Southwest Regional Meeting, American Orthopsychiatric Association, November, 1972.
33. Dingman, P. R. *Toward a workable conception of "responsibility" for the inmate of a mental institution.* Staff presentation at Grafton State Hospital, North Grafton, Massachusetts, June, 1971.
34. Fischer, R. W. Mental institutions and similar phenomena called schools. *Personnel and Guidance Journal,* 1971, **50,** 45–50.
35. Mayhon, J., Brown, L. C., Dingman, P. R., & Melancon, R. A. New Mexico's community development project, an exploration in human service delivery (Digest). *American Journal of Orthopsychiatry,* 1972, **42,** 257–259.

## Additional Works Consulted

Dingman, P. R. *Changing institutional programs for children and adolescents.* Paper presented at the Hospital Improvements Projects Committee and NIMH Staff Workshop, Washington, D.C., 1965.
Dingman, P. R., & staff. *Grafton State Hospital Proposed Program Plan for 1971–1975.* Grafton State Hospital, North Grafton, Massachusetts, 1971.
Dingman, P. R. *Toward a moratorium on referrals to children's institutions.* President's address, Section on Clinical Child Psychology, American Psychological Association, Honolulu, 1972.
Hanson, J. H., & Dingman, P. R. *Considerations in planning for children in transition.* Paper presented at Technical Assistance Project on State Operated Residential Treatment Programs for Children, Trevose, Pennsylvania, 1966.
Lion, J. R., & Pasternak, S. A. Countertransference reactions to violent patients. *American Journal of Psychiatry,* 1973, **130**(2), 207–210.

# II
## The Impact of the Closing

# 6

# The Impact of the Closing of DeWitt State Hospital

SAMUEL WEINER

Conditions that promote the closure of state hospitals for the mentally ill and mentally retarded prevail throughout the nation. Declining inpatient populations, a growing emphasis on community programs, the high overhead cost of large institutions, and the limited funds available for mental health programs make closing mental hospitals an increasingly viable alternative.

In 1969 the California Department of Mental Hygiene reported that the state would soon phase out the Modesto State Hospital. Shortly thereafter it was leaked that DeWitt State Hospital would also be phased out; moreover, it appeared that the state might completely remove itself from the direct delivery of services to the mentally ill, if not the mentally retarded. In response to this actual change in California and the possibility of similar actions in other areas of the country, Stanford Research Institute proposed a study to investigate the consequences of phasing out large, state-run mental institutions. The result of this proposal was a grant to study the consequences of the DeWitt closing, from a year before it closed to a year after the closing.

Aside from any political consequences, which might be unique to each area, there are assumed to be general economic and social impacts resulting from state hospital closings. The broad objective of this study

SAMUEL WEINER • Stanford Research Institute, Menlo Park, California 94025.

was to evaluate all of these impacts on the Auburn, California, community. The project team isolated five main areas of interest: (1) political processes affecting the decision to close DeWitt State Hospital; (2) the impact on employees; (3) the economic consequences for the community; (4) the effect on organizations and community attitudes; (5) because of budgetary limitations the fifth area, the effect on patients and treatment programs was reviewed in a fairly casual and very preliminary fashion.* This chapter presents a summary discussion of our main results.†

## The Five Areas of Concern

### Political Considerations‡

The administration of the state of California had ample reason to close DeWitt State Hospital. The hospital was originally purchased to provide a "temporary" solution to the problem of overcrowding in state hospitals. During the last several years, the problem of overcrowding had disappeared, and by 1971 DeWitt's inpatient population had declined 79% from its peak. The problem then was the increasing number of empty beds available in the hospital system. In July 1969, local programs became responsible for determining how state hospitals would be used in caring for mentally ill patients. As of July 1, 1971, the state regional centers for the mentally retarded became responsible for state hospital admissions for the retarded.

The rationale for choosing to close DeWitt included considerations of cost, physical facility, and program: (a) DeWitt was more costly than the statewide average in 17 of 23 cost centers. (b) DeWitt's total overhead could be saved by transferring patients to other hospitals and to local programs. (c) DeWitt's physical plant was unsatisfactory and unattractive. (d) Professional studies showed a low-quality treatment program. (e) Local programs were unwilling to use the hospital to the extent necessary to justify its overhead costs.

---

*Additional work was done in this area using a sample of discharged patients from Napa State Hospital. See Place, D. M., & Weiner, S. *Reentering the community: A pilot study of mentally ill patients discharged from Napa State Hospital.* Stanford Research Institute, June 1974.

†See Weiner, S. et al. *Process & impacts of a state hospital closing: The first year.* Stanford Research Institute, February 1972; and Weiner, S. et al. *Process & impacts of the closing of DeWitt State Hospital: Final report.* Stanford Research Institute, May 1973, for a more extended discussion of the issues.

‡Most of the field work concerned with the political considerations was carried out by Arthur Bolton Associates of Sacramento, California.

Although there were good reasons for closing DeWitt, the state administration apparently did not deal effectively with the political ramifications of the decision. As a result, it seemed that the political problems were handled on an ad hoc basis, creating confusion, misunderstanding, and distrust.

The problem that appeared to be of major concern when the decision to close DeWitt became final was the expected adverse effect on the community. DeWitt State Hospital was the largest single employer in Placer County, which was then in a relatively depressed economic condition. In order to overcome political pressure caused by these concerns, the state offered to turn DeWitt over to the county at no cost, providing that the county operate the hospital as a mental facility for three years. Following were the terms for negotiating the transfer of DeWitt to county operation: (a) Placer County would take over DeWitt with equipment sufficient to operate a 700-bed hospital; (b) 300 of the 700 places would be for mentally ill patients; (c) 400 beds would be for the mentally retarded, reimbursable by 50% state and 50% federal funds; and (d) The state would guarantee mentally retarded patients eligible for such reimbursement.

During the course of prolonged negotiations several inconsistencies arose. Several of the more serious, which eventually led to a breakdown in the negotiations, were:

1. In offering to transfer the operation of the hospital to Placer County, the Department of Mental Hygiene guaranteed an inpatient population of 300 mentally ill and 400 mentally retarded, a promise that could not be fulfilled under the terms of the Mental Health Act of 1968.
2. Department of Mental Hygiene representatives negotiated with Placer County representatives on the basis of full cost reimbursement for the patients "guaranteed" by the state. The administration had not authorized these terms; therefore the state would save no money with such an agreement.
3. Department representatives told Placer County that the maintenance costs of the hospital were below the state average, while the Department of Finance figures showed that they were well above the state average.
4. The date of closure was changed three times. Initially, DeWitt was to be closed July 1, 1971; then, as a result of negotiations with the county, it was postponed until July 1, 1972. In January 1971, the Department of Mental Hygiene announced that the hospital would be closed on the original date. Finally, the governor extended the closure date to March 31, 1972.

On April 12, 1970, the last patient left Modesto State Hospital. That was the first state mental hospital to be closed in California. As of March 20, 1972, the last patient left DeWitt, which, since negotiations for a county-run operation had not been fruitful, was closed shortly thereafter. The mental illness section of Agnew State Hospital was closed on June 24, 1972, and Mendocino followed on July 31 of that year.

The Reagan administration announced a plan at that time for removing the state from the operation of all its state hospitals for the mentally ill by mid-1977. A tentative schedule for closing state hospitals for the mentally ill and for adjustments in the care of the mentally retarded was released in early 1973.

These announcements led to an outcry by mental health professional and user advocate groups, which set the stage for an investigation by a newly created Senate Select Committee on Proposed Phaseout of State Hospital Services. The result of the opposition generated led to the scrapping of the formal plan to phase out hospitals for the mentally ill by 1977. A major reason for this change was the testimony in the State Senate hearings on the availability of community mental health facilities. The consensus was that most local communities did not have the facilities, personnel, or programs to provide adequate care for the patients who would be released if the state phased out its hospital programs. Nor did it appear that resources could be easily or efficiently transferred from state hospitals to community facilities. Of major concern was the shortage of locked facilities and facilities for the chronically ill in the communities.

The Brown administration is currently (as of early 1975) assessing and evaluating the consequences of previous state hospital closings before announcing its plans for the future of the California state hospital system.

## Personnel Considerations

There were two main sets of questionnaires sent out to employees. One set was mailed in mid-1971; and the second, the follow-up set, was distributed in September 1972. In 1971, 550 questionnaires were distributed to personnel who were then employed at DeWitt, and 610 questionnaires were sent to appropriate former employees of DeWitt State Hospital. Of these, 52% were returned by the employees employed at the time, and 43% were returned by the terminated employee group.

In September 1972, after the hospital was closed, questionnaires were mailed to 516 of the employees who had returned the first-year questionnaire, and who had enclosed their names and addresses. Of the 516, 270 questionnaires went to employees still employed during the 1971 mailing, and 246 went to persons terminated at DeWitt by that time. An overall return of 76% was achieved from the second mailing, 217 questionnaires were received from the group still employed in 1971 and 175 from the others.

The questionnaires were designed to elicit information on personal, occupational, and behavioral characteristics of the DeWitt employees. Data obtained from the questionnaires indicated a large percentage of the former DeWitt employees were middle-aged homeowners—about half were 50 years of age of older. Most had schooling that went only through the 12th grade; and their employment at DeWitt was generally long term—40% had been employed there for 10 years or longer. Almost half of the second year sample had been psychiatric technicians at DeWitt; only 9% said they had held such a position before working at DeWitt. Among respondents with a new job since leaving DeWitt, 24% felt the new position was better than their old one; 39% said it was worse. Seventy-three percent of the second year respondents were employed; almost 17 of the remaining 27% had left the labor force. About two-thirds who were employed had accepted the option to transfer to another Department of Mental Hygiene facility. Twenty-nine percent of those accepting the transfer went to Napa State Hospital, and another 19% went to Stockton State Hospital. About one-fourth of all respondents cited increased insecurity and loss of income as a severe hardship that they incurred because of DeWitt's being closed.

In general, second-year results indicate support of our previous findings that the expectations of employees with regard to employment and salary prospects were too pessimistic. We also found that the minimum acceptable salary for those who had been employed at DeWitt during the first-year survey had fallen sharply if they were unemployed during the second year of the study.

A random sample of approximately 10% of the respondents to the questionnaire were selected for an in-depth interview lasting about one hour. Almost all of the respondents said they would be willing to be interviewed.

Highlights of that interview are presented here.* There was a pattern of initial anxiety and then a period of denial following announcement of the closing. Once reality of the closing became too obvious to be denied, depression seemed to set in. This was followed

*See Chapter IV of the *Final Report* for a more detailed discussion.

by a significant drop in employee morale and a deterioration of the employees' attitudes toward their jobs. Although the data on this sequence of reactions are admittedly impressionistic, the sequence was repetitive enough to deserve consideration. It also appears that the closure of DeWitt, along with later closures, had a serious adverse effect on the confidence of many persons in state employment, at least in the area of mental health.

Another aspect of employee responses was the indication that most employees appeared to have a poor understanding of the reasons for closing DeWitt. Most of the persons who could articulate the official reasons rejected them, often presenting conflicting data to support their disagreement. DeWitt employees demonstrated a general ignorance of the concepts of community mental health. This seemed to add to the problem of not understanding why the hospital closed, which, in turn, must have contributed to the general hostility expressed toward its closing.

Problems related to the closing procedures appear to have included a lack of clarity about the timing of the phaseout, a lack of adequate information about transfer procedures and options, and poor communications between the hospital administration and employees regarding issues for which the employees felt they should have had more reliable information.

Psychiatric technicians are probably the class of employee most adversely affected by the closing of state hospitals. Their formal education levels are fairly low, given their salaries, and their psychiatric training is relatively limited in its applicability to other positions. The psychiatric technician probably has very limited labor market potential outside the state hospital system at pay scales comparable to those in state hospitals.

Finally, terminated employees apparently either found other work quickly (mainly through transfers), or they became part of the pool of long-term unemployed. Many of the female employees were part of the secondary labor force and dropped out of the labor market.

## Economic Considerations

In Auburn, California, and similar areas where a large state hospital like DeWitt is located there are several important considerations to note in reviewing the economic effects of the state hospital closing. First is the employment opportunities for displaced hospital staff in the immediate vicinity. Second is the distance of the facility from major labor market areas, such as is usually found in an SMSA. A third consideration is based on the belief that the greater the share of total local employment made up from the payroll of the state hospital facility, the greater the overall impact of a change in the status of that facility.

In discussing the economic impact of closing DeWitt State Hospital in the Auburn area, it must be remembered that the closure took place in what had generally been a depressed economy. Long-term declines in gold mining, lumbering, and agricultural activities were major elements in the area's general economic decline in the mid-1950s. There was some upsurge with the expansion of the space program and some public works projects, but in the late 1960s, a drastic reduction in space program spending and completion of a large water project led to another slump that has continued to the present. Somewhat offsetting the reduction in economic activity was the growth of other public works construction on water and road projects.

Into this depressed economy came the closure of DeWitt with an annual payroll of about $7.2 million. Our estimate of the direct loss to the Auburn area economy, in terms of reduced spending, came to $5.2 million. That figure consisted of $4.8 million in direct loss that DeWitt employees would probably have spent in the area, $0.17 million that the hospital itself would have spent locally, and $0.2 million that patients would have spent in the Auburn area. The indirect losses for which the project team has been able to make some reasonable estimates are from $5.2 million to $5.6 million. These losses arise from an assumed multiplier of 1 and a reduction in home-care payments over time. The assumed multiplier is an approximate but acceptable guide for an economy of the type around Auburn.

The foregoing direct and indirect monetary loss from closing DeWitt State Hospital does not appear to have had any significant adverse effect on the Auburn area economy. The economy is at least as well off now as before the closing decision was announced.

Increasing construction expenditures for the Auburn Dam and associated activities are important reasons why closing DeWitt did not have an adverse economic effect in the area. Another important consideration that probably has offset the economic effect of closing the hospital is the migration into the area of people (mostly elderly retired) who have boosted spending without adding to the unemployment problem. These people have settled in the area between Auburn and Grass Valley along Highway 49, which bordered DeWitt State Hospital.

In April 1970, a large housing condominium (Auburn Greens) opened with 125 units. The project was close to DeWitt, and many felt that because of depressed conditions and the hospital's anticipated closure, the development would have difficulty attracting occupants.

However, it was filled by late 1971, and the developer has applied for a permit to build another 214 units there. The occupants are mainly older people.

More recently there has been an increase in the level of unemployment due to the general slump in the nation's economy. The sharp drop in housing construction has led to increased unemployment in the lumber industry, and reduced freight shipments have led to some railroad connected layoffs in nearby Roseville. With all this, however, the Auburn area economy is no worse off now than it was prior to the announcement of the decision to close DeWitt State Hospital in the late 1960s.

## Community Considerations

The DeWitt State Hospital seems to have had little more than a cursory relationship with local social service agencies in the community, except for the Department of Vocational and Rehabilitation and the Alternate Care Services Unit agency. Closing DeWitt does not appear to have had a significant negative impact on any of the agencies contacted, which is consistent with the finding that it had little impact on the Auburn community in general. The only direct negative effect of the closure cited by the agencies contacted was the loss of a previously available resource. To some this meant the loss of a convenient long-term placement facility; to others it meant the loss of specific programs—for example, the adolescent treatment program and the alcoholism programs, for which no alternative local programs have been developed.

On the other hand, the closing of DeWitt stimulated the expansion of the local community mental health program. Several agencies now feel they have many more outpatient and consultation services available to them. The school system appears to have particularly benefited by the expansion of the community mental health program. Sierra View, a private contractor of mental health services, plans on increasing its involvement with local agencies.

The acquisition of the DeWitt facilities and the legislative mandates regarding its possible use have allowed the county to reduce its capital expansion plans significantly. Moreover, it has given the county the opportunity to improve facilities for local agencies and provides potential for limited growth through attracting private enterprise.

## Patient Considerations

It was generally felt by employees of the state hospital system that closing the hospital had a negative effect on patients. However, one knowledgeable professional interviewed suggested that the chronics were probably helped by the closure. Simply moving them out of their position as "institutionalized fixtures" would, it was felt, be a positive change. Others also felt that patients would benefit from the closure, especially after the initial shock of relocation or release. Unfortunately, we have not been able in this study to verify or deny either claim. The area of patient impact is clearly the one needing the most work. Our attempt to investigate this area on a very limited budget was very unsatisfactory.

We do know that released patients go into some local community. We also know that the mental health services available in different communities vary widely. From a purely quantitative view, during the past decade, outpatient admissions in all county mental health programs increased an average of almost 33% per year, while inpatient admissions increased about 21% per year over the period from 1960–1961 to 1971–1972.

Local areas face several problems in achieving an adequate level of community mental health care. One problem is the difficulty of carrying an adequate range of mental health programs. Another is the lack of "adequate" funding and the uncertainty of its flow over time.

Review of research into the closing of a large mental hospital in Canada showed that chronic psychiatric patients could be released into the community without dire effects.* However, the validity of that result depended in large part on continuity of care being available close to the released patient's residence. That continuity appears to depend on the existence of an adequate community mental health program. The case used, in Saskatchewan, involved planning by both the province and the local areas in preparing needed local programs.

## Conclusions

California has closed three state mental hospitals and the mental illness wing of another during the last three years. Moreover, other states may follow California in shifting the focus of attention to the development of community mental health facilities to take care of mental health needs. Such a reorientation will have economic, social, political, and therapeutic implications. We have attempted to deter-

*See, for example, Stewart, A., Lafave, H. G., Grunberg, F., & Herjanic, M. Problems in phasing out a large psychiatric hospital. *American Journal of Psychiatry*, July 1968, *125* (1); and Fakhruddin, A. K. M., Manjooran, A., Nair, N. P. V., & Neufeldt, A. A five-year outcome of discharged chronic psychiatric patients. *Journal of the Canadian Psychiatric Association*, December 1972, *17* (6).

mine the implications or effects that followed the closure of DeWitt State Hospital. Some of these effects are unique to the Auburn area, where DeWitt was located, or to those engaged specifically in the operations of DeWitt. Other more general consequences, given a hospital closing approach similar to that at DeWitt State Hospital, will be felt wherever a hospital is closed. The following discussion outlines these general consequences, and also offers some suggestions for mitigating their adverse effects.

## Communications

The administrative agencies carrying out the decision to phase out a mental hospital should be straightforward and unequivocal with regard to what is happening, to whom it is happening, how the various elements will be handled, and the reason why the action is being taken. Moreover, the counterarguments and doubts should be understood so they can be addressed directly. If this were done, it might lessen the high rates of denial of reality and the effects that such denial has on staff behavior.

More effective communication with hospital staff was certainly needed at DeWitt. The staff members' chosen leaders should have been brought into the closing procedure at *every stage of the process.* Employees at DeWitt did not know clearly and unequivocally why the hospital was being closed. Because of this fact, rumors abounded. For example, one rumor was that the University of California at Davis Medical School was instrumental in the decision to close DeWitt and that the reason for doing so was a desire by U. C. Davis to build up its own psychiatric unit. People who feel such rumors are of importance to the closing are less likely to accept the inevitability of the closing. They are more likely to feel that considerations such as these can be overcome by political pressure.

Denial of the reality of the closing occurred among both DeWitt and Modesto employees. Thus, it would seem that denial is a common reaction to news of a closure and that this denial will be reinforced by almost any rumor or activity that might arise. (Of course, a statement concerning future closings in California, were it to be released now, would have an effect different from the same statement released with regard to the DeWitt closing. Whatever else might result from such a statement, it is hard to imagine interested parties denying the reality of future state hospital closings.)

The statements of many employees indicate that after closure is announced, staff members begin to spend a significant amount of time discussing the closure and the associated rumors. It would be useful if the time so consumed could be devoted to structured discussions with hospital administrators and Department of Mental Hygiene representatives to consider aspects of the closure that are relevant to employees.

## Staff Anxiety, Patient Care, and Carry-Over of Feelings

How much patient anxiety is caused by the contagion of staff anxiety over closing a hospital? This question seems particularly cogent since the psychiatric technicians, who are the staff members in closest contact with patients, seem to be the group of employees whose own security is most threatened by the reality of closure.

Further, the interviews conducted suggest the relevance of two other questions: Are patient attitudes toward transfer affected by employee reactions to the knowledge the hospital is closing? Do employees who transfer to other state hospitals carry with them, and maintain, a negative attitude toward their job as a result of personal problems and difficulties resulting from the closure? Although our observations were limited, impressions came through clearly enough to suggest that something should be done during the closure period to maintain better control of employee response, especially as it affects patients.

The other issue, carry-over and continuation of negative reaction, is much more difficult to pinpoint. What we found to be true for the DeWitt personnel in this regard has surely been conditioned by later developments concerning future closures. During the first year, we found that negative attitudes among those involved in the closing process were fairly pervasive. During the second year, we found a remarkable similarity in the statements of employees, especially with regard to attitudes toward the closure of DeWitt and criticisms of the closing process. The intensity of employee feelings had diminished very little, and, in some cases, had increased.

Without a doubt, the closure of DeWitt represented a severe hardship to many employees and created a life crisis for a significant number of employees. In several cases reported, the loss of staff morale suffered during the closure seems to have carried over to transfer jobs. (This did not appear to be true for those who found employment outside of the Department of Mental Hygiene.)

Clearly, the state must be better prepared to cope with the problems of displaced personnel, so as to minimize some of the problems that will arise. One general DeWitt staff complaint which could easily have been avoided was that there was insufficient information from the hospital administration about transfer options, and about when individuals would be asked to transfer. This left people uncertain about their future employment, and certainly contributed to the general state of anxiety. A specific factor that caused considerable resentment in both the DeWitt and Modesto closures was the opening up of highly desirable Stockton State Hospital positions after transfers were well under way, i.e., when it was too late for many to change direction.

## Timing the Phaseout

The length of time over which the closing of DeWitt took place had some negative effects, but the gradual nature of the closure had some positive effects as well. The main benefit was that it allowed some adjustments to be made that would not have been possible in a short time. For example, at the time of the announcement of the phaseout decision, it was felt that the economic impact would be serious. However, over time, other factors came into play and mitigated the expected effects on the Auburn area economy.

Members of the Overall Economic Development Committee for the city of Auburn felt that because the county fought to keep DeWitt open, it gained almost a 2-year extension of the closing. Over this 21- to 24-month period, adjustments were made in the area which would have been less likely if the facility had been closed soon after the decision was made. There is some trade-off here between time needed for necessary readjustments and employee anxiety that might be caused by the arguments put forth to slow down (ostensibly to prevent) closure.

## Positive Effects on the Community

One important effect was the activity of groups that came together, first to try to save the hospital (prevent the closing), and then to develop alternative uses of the new county facility. These groups were a positive force for constructive change in the community. They brought together people who under other circumstances might not have worked together. From looking at such narrow issues as alternative uses of DeWitt facilities, they became involved in larger issues of community concern.

Another positive effect has been the growth of the county mental health facilities. This also received stimulation from the closing of DeWitt. Although the closing alone was not the only force to create this change, the nature of this crisis was one of the key factors in bringing it about. The local community mental health program in the Auburn area has improved significantly in the past year, and it now appears to be on the way toward meeting local needs. Much of the improvement has occurred since the intervention of Sierra View,* and it seems reasonable to expect continued improvement of local mental health services. Whether it will be possible, given current funding problems, to provide the range of needed services for different patient groups remains to be seen. However, the problem of what facilities the community should develop for chronic patients must be faced. Given the drain on resources involved in care for chronics, some hard thinking and innovation are needed in this area. Since the decision to close all state hospitals for the mentally ill by 1977 was scrapped, the problem is not as critical as it once appeared. However, the Brown administration will have to look into the alternatives available if community care is to be a viable alternative.

## Aggregate Effects Versus Individual Effects

In the aggregate, it appears that the negative economic impact of the DeWitt closure has been more than offset by other economic forces at work in the area. However, this is certainly not true for many individuals displaced or affected by the closure. For one thing, employment at DeWitt was an important second source of income for many families. Loss of this source was especially harmful where the other income came from seasonal work. Moreover, many of the second-income earners were secondary workers who could not relocate; these tended to drop out of the labor force.

There are indications that employees who suffered this most enduring negative effect of closure were older persons less than 10 years away from retirement. Because of the handicap of age, these employees had fewer alternative employment options open to them and felt forced to accept a transfer. These were often employees with the most years of service within the Department of Mental Hygiene. Because of their age and general orientation to rural living, the need to relocate was much more of a hardship. It seems reasonable to suggest, therefore, that retirement options be made more liberal or flexible for employees over a certain age and with a given number of years of state service.

Another example of individual effects that are lost in aggregate results is exemplified by the following quote from a returned question-

---

*Sierra View is an affiliate of Kings View Hospital in Tulare County, California. Kings View is a health care organization developed by Mennonites. They also administer two county health care programs in the Fresno, California, area.

naire: "The real blow came when, after my termination, the Welfare Department notified me that, since my five years of retirement benefits are now available to me, they represent personal property over what is allowed and this disqualified us for further benefits." This decision stopped the supplemental welfare checks (both husband and wife were unemployed) as well as availability of Medi-Cal benefits. Retirement benefits, even if available earlier than actual retirement, should be seen as an available resource only during retirement.

Although it may be difficult to structure general provisions to take care of special cases, we should be aware of individual problems. In planning for a closure, the state should set up a mechanism whereby special problems are brought to the attention of knowledgeable parties and, where possible, corrective measures are taken.

### Cost/Patient Ratios and the Assessment of Patient Impact

A large reduction in the state hospital population followed development of community centers and the widespread use of psychotropic drugs, along with financial inducement offered by the state to keep patients in the local community.

Reducing the patient population in any institution such as a mental hospital will undoubtedly lead to an increase in the cost/patient ratio for those remaining. The extent to which unit cost increases will depend upon the extent to which operating costs can be reduced as patient load decreases. In most cases, operating costs fall very slowly, if at all. At best they usually do not drop until a significant length of time after the patient load is reduced. Consequently, cost/patient ratios invariably increase, usually fairly sharply, as patient load falls.

As a result of the rise in cost/patient ratios, supporting agencies (usually government organizations) "find" that the institution is no longer feasible to maintain from an economic point of view. This has certainly been true for mental hospitals. In the final report, we showed that the estimated cost/patient day at DeWitt, as of January 31, 1971, was $7.46, whereas the statewide average was only $5.60 per patient day. However, DeWitt's inpatient population had fallen to a low of 899 as an average for 1970, which meant that the population as of January 31, 1971, was probably around 700 (as late as 1965 the average inpatient population at DeWitt was over 2,000 patients). Therefore, the fact that DeWitt cost/patient ratios were higher than the statewide average in 1971 is hardly surprising. More surprising is the fact that the difference was not greater than that shown above.

Cost considerations are important, but they should be viewed in

terms of alternatives. The issue really is whether the total social benefits, including the monetary ones, among different methods of serving
patient population are greater under the noninstitutional arrangement
of patient care. Crucial elements in determining such benefits are an
assessment of the relative benefit to patients of being kept in the
community versus being placed in a state institution, and an assessment of the effect either alternative is likely to have on the community.
Unfortunately, reliable indications of patient impact are most difficult
to obtain.*

An assessment of the impact on patients is needed for another
reason. Employees in the second-year sample, as well as those interviewed a year earlier, continually remarked on the effect closing the
hospital had on patients and on seeing the same patients in other
hospitals in a deteriorated condition. The frequency and sincerity of
these expressions of concern suggests that a serious study of the effects
of hospital closure on patients would be most appropriate. Not only
would such a study provide valuable information that could be used to
minimize negative effects on patients, but it could also address itself to
concerns of employees which seem to affect their attitudes toward
transfer and their general level of morale.

## Changing Attitudes Toward Closure

A follow-up of community attitudes a year after the DeWitt State
Hospital was closed indicated a significant reduction in the intensity of
negative attitudes. There was less change, however, in the direction of
attitudes (e.g., negative to positive). It appears that persons whose
opposition to the closure was based primarily on general local concerns
(economic decline, lack of services, etc.) were most likely to express a
change in attitude when their fears were not realized. Changes in
persons with negative attitudes related to personal concerns ("my business," "my job," "my home," etc.) also depended on actual outcomes.
Persons least likely to experience a change of attitude were those whose
opposition was based on principle, e.g., resistance to the concept of
community mental health. This latter group might represent a potential
target population toward which educational efforts might be directed.
Our study of the attitudes of hospital employees suggests that a hospital
closure should be accompanied by a concerted effort to educate the staff
regarding the theory of community mental health, including support-

*However, see the chapters by E. W. Markson and J. H. Cumming, as well as that by R. A.
Marlowe, in this volume.

ing documentation. Our survey of general community attitudes also seems to suggest that similar measures should be undertaken on a broader public scale.

## Closing a State Hospital: Issues of Major Concern

The protracted negotiations between Placer County and the state, and the denouement when the Department of Mental Hygiene announced its intention to pay the county for patient care at about half the rate quoted throughout the negotiations, appear to have been the source of much hard feeling. During the second year of this study, the subject of the negotiations was often raised by persons interviewed. People in the Auburn community and in Sacramento still rankled over what they perceived as "shabby" treatment by the state.

A reporter for the *Auburn Journal* summarized: "Nobody gave a straight answer." He included the state senator and assemblyman in this comment, who, he felt, were playing another political game with the issue.*

A legislative committee consultant who had monitored the County-State negotiations in 1971 as representative of the Department of Finance said: "In retrospect, the dire effects were caused largely by the irrational political situation. When the Governor and others use the closure to play political games, pre-planning will have little or no results. It was misleading for the State to negotiate with a small, poor county like Placer to assume the operation of DeWitt."†

Placer County Supervisor Ray Thompson, who participated in the County-State negotiations, had a more charitable explanation for the course of events: "There were so many cross signals. There were no firm, set rules for anyone in General Services of DMH to negotiate from. Somebody kept changing the ground rules in the Governor's office. People said things in good faith, but things kept changing."‡

Several general probem areas to be considered in any closing were brought out in our interviews: timing, communication, and financing. On the timing issue, one knowledgeable participant in the state legislative process said: "To lessen the impact of closing, set plans in motion far enough in advance to smooth out closure, reduce or close down admissions and transfer gradually; prepare patients well in advance, and lengthen the time between announcing and accomplishing the closing.

*Joe Carroll, *Auburn Journal*, February 23, 1973.
†Stanley Lena, Assembly Committee on Social Welfare, Interview, February 6, 1973.
‡Ray Thompson, Supervisor, Placer County, Interview, March 20, 1973.

"It is probably not possible to close a hospital without having some political and economic impact, especially in small counties where hospitals play a major role."*

The communication issue also bears on the timing issue. Although the time that elapsed from the announcement to the actual closing of DeWitt was 28 months, the "mixed signals" clouded this fact. Two comments suggesting a better approach were the following.

> To prevent adverse reactions in further state hospital closures, there should be full disclosure when a hospital is to be closed; time should be given for the community to get used to the idea. However, it is probably not possible to fully prevent adverse reactions. Community planning groups make reports of pros and cons which sometimes do nothing more than stir up the people.†
>
> The DeWitt closing was not publicly stated until after rumors had floated around. Instead, the announcement should have been made after first explaining to parents why the transfer was necessary. Advocate organizations should have been brought in on the ground floor.‡

The financial aspects of the situation were illuminated by the staff of the County Supervisors Association. The problem of making "the dollar flow with the patient" has plagued the mental health system since the implementation of the 90–10 state–county matching formula in 1969. At legislative hearings, local program directors complained that they would accept responsibility for released patients but would not receive the money that they were saving the state. Now local programs receive the $15/day "bounty," but apparently the funding lag occurring with hospital closures is adding a new strain: "There is not a smooth flow of dollars from the State to the counties. The State tries to have counties implement programs without any 'prepping' costs; money is available after the fact so counties have to put up the money first, then be reimbursed later.

"The question is whether or not the counties will be able to afford long-term care. I suggest that counties be given money at the time the hospital closes so they will be able to afford to pick up some of the hospital staff immediately.§

---

*Steven Thompson, Assembly Committee on Ways and Means.
†Dennis Amundson, Administrative Assistant to Assemblyman Frank Lanterman.
‡William Green, Executive Director, California Association for the Retarded.
§Dale Wagerman, Health and Welfare Coordinator, County Supervisors Association of California, Interview, March 5, 1973.

# 7

# When They Closed the Doors at Modesto*

ROBERTA A. MARLOWE

## Introduction

One of the patients in my study group spent the major portion of her time at Modesto sitting mute in a chair by the office pleating her dress; she would start from the hem and work up to her stomach, then smooth down the material to begin again. In a psychiatric summary this might be referred to as compulsive ritualistic behavior. Immediately upon entering a convalescent hospital, she located, cornered, and seduced a not unwilling male—in full view of her roommate and staff and patients who happened to pass by the open door. When we studied her a year after relocation, she (1) had learned to close the door, (2) availed herself of a variety of additional social and recreational activities, and (3) no longer pleated her clothing.

Another patient spent most of her time at Modesto cleaning, mopping, helping serve food, caring for less capable patients, and in other ways acting as an assistant to the staff. She was highly sociable,

*Derived from the study, *Modesto relocation project: Social–psychological consequences of relocating geriatric state hospital patients*, R. A. Marlowe, Principal Investigator; Project 1–60, Bureau of Research, Department of Mental Hygiene, State of California, 1969–1972.

ROBERTA A. MARLOWE • Department of Health of the State of California, Sacramento, California.

extremely verbal, independent, bossy, critical, alert, and paranoid. When studied a year later, she spent all of her time sitting in a chair; she refused to work, rarely spoke to anyone, and gave the appearance of lethargy and unawareness. When interviewed, she explained that she was "here for a rest" and hoped to return to her home at Modesto.

Both of these ladies were over 65 years of age and long-time residents in the state hospital community. Together, in their diametrically opposed outcomes, as in their very existence, they exemplify the dilemma which is the subject of this volume: What should be done about social policy? What is the preferred pattern of service for individuals identified as mentally ill at this time and in this place? Others have written about this question from the perspective of what could or should happen in terms of state plans. Still others have written on alternatives to state hospitals. There *are* alternatives; there always have been, and very probably some of them will prove superior to the patterns we have thus far developed for this group. However, there is another problem. A lot of human beings are currently in state hospitals. The decisions made will have a profound impact upon their lives.

Next to the question of what is the best societal plan for the delivery of mental health services, is another important problem: the consequence of changing the pattern of service delivery to those who are long-time recipients of service in the current system. This question has meaning not only in terms of the lives of those affected but also in terms of what their experiences can tell us about the characteristics which must be developed in future systems if they are to be any less of an evil than our current or historical patterns.

The elderly are star candidates for relocation when state hospitals are phased down or closed. In state hospitals, as elsewhere, the treatment of the elderly is likely to be viewed as professionally unrewarding and of low social consequence. Accordingly, while the allocation of *treatment* resources to this group is low, state hospitals tend to collect increasing numbers of elderly persons who consume larger and larger portions of the space and operating budgets of such institutions. In 1965, nearly 30% of the residents of California state hospitals were age 65 or older.[1]

At the same time, the elderly, long-term resident of a state hospital is unlikely to have a family to whom he may be returned, he is likely to have lost whatever vocational skills he might once have possessed, and he is likely to be lacking many of the rudimentary personal and social skills necessary for caring for his own needs. For this kind of individual, the hospital often represents the only home, the only support system, the only social context which he has known in years.

An increasing body of gerontological research attests to the fact that the movement of such persons cannot be done without risk: Aldrich and Mendkoff, Jasnau, Markus, Aleksandrowics, Killian, Lieberman, and others have all reported increased rates of death and/or of physical or psychological deterioration following the relocation of the aged.[2]

The research in this report addresses the question of the consequences to elderly individuals of their relocation from a state hospital. Three main issues will be touched on:

1. What happened to the elderly inhabitants of a state hospital after relocation: Where did they go, did they survive, did the survivor experience changes in condition or level of functioning following relocation?
2. To whom did these outcomes occur: What kinds of individuals experienced what kinds of outcomes, what factors provide the best explanation for these outcomes?
3. To what kinds of places were the patients relocated: Is there a relationship between individual outcome and environment, what kinds of environments were the most and the least enhancing for what kinds of individuals?

## Setting and Study Group

The hospital which provided the subjects for our investigation was Modesto State Hospital, the first in the California system to be closed. Between September 1969 and April 1970, 1,100 residents of this hospital were relocated; approximately 40% of these patients were age 65 or older. Our study group of 429 comprised 93% of those who were 65 years of age or older. We defined age 65 as anyone who was, or who would be, age 65 as of November 30, 1969; additionally, we excluded a few patients who had been hospital residents for less than 90 days, as our interest was in the long-term resident of state hospitals (only 9 patients were so excluded). Our criteria embraced 461 patients as of September 1, 1969; of these, 23 died before they could be relocated, 3 were transferred in acute medical emergency, and 6 were lost through administrative confusion; the resultant 429 constituted our study group.

Modesto was unique in the California state hospital system in that it not only had a higher than average concentration of the elderly—40% as opposed to 20% in the system as a whole at the time[3]—but it also had a very high proportion of individuals who had been hospitalized 20 years or more; 72% of our study group had been hospitalized for this length of time.*

As could be expected within a group which had been hospitalized for this length of time, our patients were quite debilitated in many spheres. A quarter of the group was bedridden or could ambulate only with physical or mechanical assistance. Sixty percent needed physical assistance or considerable individual prompting to accomplish self-care. Less than half remained continent at all times. Sixty percent were either functionally nonverbal or had never been heard to speak more than a short sentence. A third were foreign born. Half of our patients were diagnosed as schizophrenic and a third carried the designation of chronic brain syndrome, primarily from senility or cerebral arteriosclerosis. The most common psychiatric symptoms in the group were those related to withdrawal—forgetfulness, confusion, inability to keep to a time schedule. Half of our patients literally spent all of their time sitting, rising only for meals or to go to the bathroom.

Although our study group as a whole could be placed at the debilitated end of several continua, there was, nevertheless, a good deal of heterogeneity within the group. When the patients' prerelocation characteristics were analyzed by a clustering technique,[4] seven discrete patient "types" were identified:

*Total Care Patients* (16%). Extremely physically incapacitated individuals who were confined to their beds, suffering from numerous serious illnesses, and who were totally dependent upon skilled nursing care for life sustenance; they tended to have been hospitalized for two years or less and to carry diagnoses of chronic brain syndrome.

*The Institutionalized* (16%). Persons with minimal ambulatory abilities who could care for a few of their own needs but who had become functionally debilitated and physically ill after extremely long periods of hospitalization; they tended to be in poor contact with reality and to exhibit few psychiatric symptoms other than confusion.

*The Alert Physically Ill* (16%). Alert and sociable individuals who cared for many of their own needs but who suffered from multiple and severe somatic ailments which limited their ability to participate in the ward routine and which gave them a very poor prognosis.

*The Healthy Out-of-Contact* (17%). Physically healthy, ambulatory individuals who could care for most of their own needs, but who were

*Department of Mental Hygiene, 1965.[1] Both of these differences were a function primarily of the fact that Modesto had been opened as a "temporary" transfer facility which was designed to alleviate the overcrowded conditions in other hospitals after World War II. Eighty-three percent of my study group came by transfer from another hospital.

only minimally responsive to their environments and nearly totally nonsociable.

The Disturbed (8%). Long-hospitalized individuals who were extremely deficient in a functional sense, who manifested many psychiatric symptoms and who were neither responsive nor sociable.

The Normals (17%). Persons who were not debilitated in any sphere; they were alert, responsible, sociable, physically healthy, functionally proficient, and displayed no psychiatric symptoms.

The Elite (11%). Highly sociable and responsive individuals who were physically healthy, highly independent in self-care, and who functioned as "ward bosses" or "patient aides" on their hospital units; they were differentiated from the Normals chiefly in their relatively high manifestation of psychiatric symptomatology.

## Method

In this study we used a before–after design which encompassed both the study group and an unrelocated control group. Since we were interested in change, as well as in mortality, as a consequence of relocation, a considerable amount of time was expended in assessing the characteristics of the patients *prior* to their relocation from Modesto. A combination of data-gathering techniques were used, with a heavy reliance placed upon the direct observation of patients in their home units;* these data were supplemented by an extensive interview with the staff members who knew the patient most thoroughly, by an interview with the patient whenever possible, and by a review of the patient's hospital records. Ratings of "patient characteristics" were made on the basis of data from all of these sources. Patients were followed up between eleven and thirteen months after relocation, and a similar combination of data-gathering tools were used in their new environments.

So that we could assess the rates of mortality and of change which might be expected to occur in a population of this type which did *not*

---

*Although the observational technique (13 hours per patient in his home unit, encompassing the patient's day from arising to bedtime) was expensive in both time and resources, it allowed us to (1) collect comparable data on all patients regardless of cognitive condition or verbal proclivity, (2) compensate for inadequate staff information, of which there was a great deal, (3) examine the way in which the patient fitted into the social system of his home unit, gaining insight into the roles which normally were performed by the patient, and (4) develop a thorough picture of the patient which would be especially useful in assessing change after relocation.

undergo the relocation process, a control group of 100 individuals was selected from another state hospital in the system.* A stratified random sampling technique was used to select these patients; age, sex, length of hospitalization, and a composite measure of self-care ability were used as selection criteria. Data-gathering techniques identical to those for the study group were used on this sample, and they also were studied at two points in time, 12 months apart.

Because we were interested in determining the influence of environment on the outcome of relocation, both the pre- and the postrelocation environments were assessed. Along with structural or formal characteristics—size, staff–patient ratio, patterns of ownership and control—elements of what may be called social–psychological millieu or institutional environment were measured by means of interviews with staff and through structured ratings based upon observation.

## Findings

### Where Did They Go?

While large numbers of Modesto's younger patients were released to the care of relatives, or discharged directly, only *two* of our elderly study group were returned to their families. Nearly half of the study group was placed in some kind of community residential facility for the aged—nursing homes, convalescent hospitals, rest or board-and-care homes. The other half was transferred to other state hospitals in the system. However, between relocation and our follow-up one year later, nearly half of the patients who had been transferred to other state hospitals were also placed in community facilities. Only *three* persons were returned to hospitals from the community during this time period. In all, 69% of the study group was placed out of state hospitals during the year.

As an attempt was made to return the patients to their counties of origin, the community facilities which housed these patients were scattered all over the state. One hundred and forty-two different community facilities and 38 different state hospital units accommodated our

---

*This hospital was selected because information provided by the Bureau of Biostatistics of California's Department of Mental Hygiene indicated that it best matches Modesto in terms of its proportion of the long-term elderly and in the kinds of programs which it offered its elderly residents. This expectation of similarity was well justified as the controls matched the Modesto population on 31 of 35 dimensions, despite the use of primarily demographic variables as selection criteria.

patients.* Sixty percent of the placed patients were located in nursing homes, 19% were located in convalescent hospitals of 100 beds or more, and 21% were housed in rest home or board and care facilities.†

Only *one* patient, out of the 429, remained out of an institution for the entire year. Our first conclusion, therefore, is that, at least for this particular group of elderly individuals, hospital closure meant movement from one institutional setting to another; in no real sense can this be termed a "return to the community."

## Did They Survive?

By the one-year follow-up, 78 (or 18%) of the patients in our study group were dead. To put this 18% figure in perspective, two sets of baseline mortality rates are available for comparison. First, in the four years prior to the closure of the hospital, an average mortality rate of 10.7% was found for patients of this age and length of hospitalization. ‡ Second, in the control group of highly comparable but nonrelocated individuals, only 5% died during the year. By either of these indices, therefore, one must conclude that relocation did have a heightening effect upon mortality: Two to three times as many patients died as could have been expected to die in the absence of relocation.

This finding is quite compatible with the results of previous investigations of postrelocation mortality. A review of the literature reveals that the highest postrelocation mortality rates were found under conditions similar to those experienced by the Modesto patients: "Forced" or nonvoluntary relocation, brought about by administrative decisions to close or to reorganize facilities, universally produces higher mortality rates than does the more voluntary movement of elderly individuals such as occurs in geriatric discharge programs.

## Did They Change?

The answer to this question also is in the affirmative: The effects of relocation were not confined to mortality. Change was assessed by means of a comparison of pre- and postrelocation scores, as well as by

---

*Of the 142 community facilities, 46 were rest homes or board-and-care homes, 67 were nursing homes, and 29 were convalescent hospitals.

†A nominal classification of care facilities with respect to size and self-definition were used for the study. Family care homes (1–5), small board-and-care (6–15), large board-and-care or rest homes (16–35), small nursing homes (under 70), large nursing homes (70–99), and convalescent hospitals (100 or more) were distinguished.

‡For the four years prior to closure (fiscal years 1967–1970), the rates were 12.7%, 11.0%, 9.5%, and 9.6% respectively.

direct ratings made by the observer-interviewers, and was measured in the four areas of physical condition, mental or psychiatric status, level of awareness, and social behavior.*

Of the surviving patients,† 159 (or 46%) deteriorated, 103 (or 29%) remained unchanged, and 87 (or 25%) improved following relocation. Half of the deteriorated patients and 40% of the improved patients changed in *more than one* of the four substantive areas.

In contrast, change in the control group was of a lesser magnitude and occurred in different areas: Control patients tended to change only in one realm, and these changes tended to occur primarily in the areas of physical and mental status; very few changes occurred in the social behavior or awareness areas. Modesto patients, on the other hand, not only tended to experience multiple changes, they much surpassed the control group in changing in the realms of awareness and of social behavior.

We must conclude that relocation had both enhancing and deleterious consequences for these patients. Although certain changes, particularly of a physical or psychiatric nature, may be expected in an aged state hospital population such as this, the stresses and opportunities attendant upon relocation increased this downhill progression for some patients and completely reversed it for others. Our data indicate that, while many more patients deteriorated markedly than probably would have in the absence of relocation, another group experienced improvement in their status or condition that also would not have occurred had they remained in their familiar environments.

## To Whom Did These Outcomes Occur?

*Death*. As has been found by other investigators,[5] mortality tends to be highly related to the patient's physical and cognitive condition prior to relocation.‡ The highest death rate was found in Total Care

---

*Multiple variables were used to determine change in each area. Only when the scores consistently were in a given direction was an outcome of change received by a patient. Where the various scores contradicted one another, entire case records were reviewed. Thus, the changes had to be considerable, and visible, to accord the patient an outcome of change.

†Two patients were not followed up. One was living on his own in a skid row tenement, the other was "lost" after going AWOL from his rest home with a broken arm. The first was reported by his sister as "doing fine"; the second could not be traced.

‡A multivariate analysis of variance indicated that the variables of Functional Capacity ($F$ =18.33, $p < .0001$), Physical Health ($F$ =12.67, $p < .0001$), Awareness ($F$ =7.04, $p < .0001$), and Social Behavior ($F$ =4.46, $p < .0001$) were, respectively, best able to predict death outcomes. Environmental factors were largely irrelevant in prediction equations for death.

group, where 47% did not survive. The Alert Physically Ill, with 28% dead, and the Institutionalized, with 19%, displayed the next highest mortality rates. These three groups rated lowest of the seven on all of our measures of physical condition. At the other extreme, very low death rates, 4% and 6% respectively, were found among the Elite and Normal groups, both, it will be recalled, composed of individuals who were physically healthy, functionally proficient, and highly aware of and responsive to their surroundings. Deaths in the two remaining groups fell between these extremes.

One must conclude, therefore, that hospital closure and forced relocation are (1) likely to increase mortality rates, and (2) especially likely to produce death among those who were in fragile physical and/or cognitive condition prior to the move.

*Change.* Turning to the characteristics of the persons who changed, a pattern emerges which is very different from the one we have just discussed. Whereas physical and cognitive condition were the best predictors of death, with those in the worst condition most likely to succumb, these factors were only marginally related to change outcomes.* In fact, in the group as a whole, those in the worst general condition were the *least* likely to change: Both deteriorated and improved patients were in better condition prior to the move than those who remained stable. The control group, on the other hand, followed a more traditional or expected pattern, with deteriorations occurring among the least adequate, and improvements among the most adequate, patients. This suggests, first, that many of the patients who died might only have experienced a relatively "normal" regression in condition if they had not been relocated, and second, that many of our deteriorated patients may have been expected to remain unchanged, or even to improve, in the absence of the relocation experience.

Our second major finding in the area of the prediction of change is that very few variables relating to patient characteristics—"person" variables—differentiated those who deteriorated from those who improved. Basically, they were the same kinds of people.†This was true

---

*Fs of 2.94 ($p <.01$), .62 ($p <.6$), and 3.14 ($p <.003$) were found, by multivariate analysis of variance, in the deteriorated/no change contrasts. Comparable $F$ and $p$ levels were found when the improved patients were contrasted with the stable ones. For both sets of contrasts, environmental variables were far superior to these in predicting outcomes—all environmental variables were at the level of $p <.0001$.

†A Discriminate Function Analysis performed on the deteriorated and improved groups revealed only three "person" variables on which the groups were significantly different: Sociability, Degree of Interaction with Staff, and Verbal Ability. All of these were at a much lower level of significance than the majority of "environmental" variables which differentiated the groups.

whether we examined the study group as a whole or the various patient "types" individually.

Differential rates of change, however, were found *between* the several patient groups. Along with the Total Care Patients, of whom 83% remained unchanged, the Institutionalized, the Healthy Out-of-Contact, and the Alert Physically Ill groups all had more than 50% of their members in the unchanged category following relocation. All three also had low rates (less than 20%) of improvement, with the remainder deteriorating. The *highest* rates of deterioration were found among the groups which were physically, cognitively, and socially capable: Nearly 70% of the Elites and 50% of the Normals experienced deterioration following relocation.

## The Influence of Environment

The relationship between outcome and environment is a strong one. As was mentioned earlier, very few "person" variables differentiated the improved and deteriorated patients. What *did* differentiate these two groups was the kind of environment manifested by the facilities or units to which they were relocated. Basically, the two groups went to vastly different kinds of environments. By environmental "differences" here, I am referring not to formal kinds or types of facilities nor to the structural characteristics of the institutions involved. Rather, I am referring to those aspects of an organization which influence the *quality of life* experienced by the resident: expectations for his behavior, attitudes held about him, the kind of treatment he receives from staff, and the nature of his relationships with other residents. On these dimensions, from the perspective of patient outcome, equally "good" and "bad" environments were located in nursing homes, in convalescent hospitals, in board-and-care homes, and in state hospitals.

Briefly, those who improved went to environments which (1) maximized resident autonomy by allowing residents some control over their own lives, (2) encouraged the treatment of residents in a personalizing, rather than in a dehumanizing, manner, (3) did not foster unnecessary dependency among residents, (4) had very little tolerance for deviant behavior, rather, expected reasonably "normal" performance from residents, (5) made some attempt to integrate its residents into the community outside of the facility or unit, and (6) encouraged social interaction among residents. Those who deteriorated tended to go to environments which rated the opposite on these several dimensions.

Further, improved patients were treated with a great deal of warmth and personalization; those who deteriorated received little of either. Attitudes toward the improved patients were highly positive, toward the deteriorated very negative. While those who deteriorated were expected to behave in a docile, passive fashion, no such expectations developed upon those who improved. And, finally, despite the lack of real differences between the groups, improved patients were viewed as more cognitively intact, relative to others in their facilities, than were the deteriorated patients.

As a group, these variables speak to the issue of the normalization of, and independence in, behavior. Facilities which encouraged residents to be independent in decision making, in use of time and space, in trying out of skills, which encouraged a "noninstitutional" pattern of relationships and activities inside and outside of the facility, and which discouraged deviant performance, were highly appropriate and beneficial to our patients. Such expectations provided a context within which growth could occur and which, indeed, encouraged development. Given the similarities between the improved and deteriorated patients, it is likely that those who deteriorated had an equal *capacity* for responding favorably to positive environmental influences. Denied these favorable conditions, this group responded with a withdrawal and a disintegration which placed them in our deteriorated category.

During the past year, I have been developing a typology of environments on the basis of the environmental dimensions which have just been mentioned. Used in conjunction with the patient typology, such a classification system allows us to address the question of "person–environment fit": What particular types of environments are most conducive to positive outcomes for what particular kinds of patients? Although I have not completed this analysis, a few highlights may serve to illustrate the general direction.

For patients in good condition on most dimensions (Elite, Normals), a challenging environment, one which asked more of them than they were accustomed to giving, appeared to be necessary. Additionally, as most of these patients had viable roles and high status positions at Modesto, environments which provided *substitutes* for these roles and positions were conducive to improvement outcomes. The majority of the Elite group was not fortunate enough to find environments of this kind.

For those in moderate health and/or cognitive condition (Alert Physically Ill, Healthy Out-of-Contact), a combination of challenging and supportive/encouraging environmental characteristics seem most appropriate. These patients tend to have formed relationships and attachments in their Modesto units, but not to have occupied high status positions. To the extent that the new environments encouraged new relationships, new learning experiences, or new roles, these patients did well; where such encouragements were lacking, or where the environment responded negatively to them (i.e., with restraints, drugs), they deteriorated.

For the physically and cognitively limited (Institutionalized, Disturbed), deteriorations appear to be a function of normal physiological processes, of trauma associated with the move itself, and of the loss of whatever minimal attachments had been developed at Modesto. The issue with this group was not the challenging nature of the environment but, rather, the amount of individual care, attention, and encouragement received by the patient.

## Conclusion

Relocation was dangerous for a majority of the patients: Deaths were increased, there was a high rate of deterioration, many patients were sent to environments which lacked the basic necessities for a decent life. Some patients were lucky; they were sent to environments which facilitated the maintenance of their prerelocation condition or even the growth or enhancement of attributes which had atrophied through desuetude.

If the decision is made to close state hospitals, some increase in death and deterioration is inevitable. Highly fragile individuals simply cannot withstand the physical or psychological assault entailed in such moves. Much of the deterioration, however, can be eliminated. This may be done by attempting to match the needs of the patient with the character of the facility to which he is sent. And the character of the facility, in my data, appears to be most determined by the attitudes toward people, and toward the elderly, which are held by *care level* staff. Some really ingenious responses to patient need were contrived by the aides and psychiatric technicians whom we studied: Modesto patients were placed together so that each had a thread of continuity after relocation; even severely limited patients were helped when they were encouraged to relate, in a caring or mothering fashion, to others *less* capable than themselves; patients who, at Modesto, made a nuisance of themselves playing in water were given the job of washing windows or walks; high-status patients were accorded the deference which they expected and were given responsibilities which supported such statuses.

These all are little things, but they imply a knowledge of patient needs and a willingness to run an organization at, perhaps, less than top efficiency but in service of the primary objective of patient care—attributes which, literally, made the difference between progression and retrogression to our patients.

In my current research, I am just beginning to explore the factors which produce attitudes of this sort. Staff–patient ratios, facility size, presence of psychiatric services, patterns of ownership or control, physical attractiveness, arrangements or resources—all of these appear *unrelated* to quality of the environment. At this point, I can only say that the kinds of attitudes which produce quality environments are not restricted to "community facilities" or to state hospitals. Enhancing and deleterious environments were found in both.

## References

1. Department of Mental Hygiene, State of California. Statistical report of the Department of Mental Hygiene, hospitals for the mentally ill and mentally retarded, June 30, 1965, p. 38.
2. Aldrich, C. K., & Mendkoff, E. Relocation of the aged and disabled: A mortality study. *Journal of the American Geriatrics Society*, 1963, **11**, 105–194. Aleksandrowics, D. Fire and its aftermath on a geriatric ward. *Bulletin of the Menninger Clinic*, 1961, **25**, 23–32. Jasnau, K. F. Individualized versus mass transfer of nonpsychotic geriatric patients from the mental hospitals to nursing homes, with special reference to death rate. *Journal of the American Geriatrics Society*, 1967, **15**(3), 280–284. Killian, E. Effect of geriatric transfer on mortality rates. *Social Work*, January 1970, **15**(1), 19–26. Markus, E., Blenkner, M., & Downs, T. The impact of relocation upon mortality rates of institutionalized aged persons. *Journal of Gerontology*, 1971, **26**, 537–541. Miller, D., & Lieberman, M. A. The relationship of affect state adaptive reactions to stress. *Journal of Gerontology*, 1965, **20**, 492–497.
3. Bureau of Biostatistics, State of California. *California Data*, Statistical Bulletin #4, September 1, 1970.
4. Try, B. C., Tyron, R. C., & Bailey, D. E. *Cluster analysis*. New York: McGraw-Hill, 1970.
5. Goldfarb, A. I. The evaluation of geriatric patients following treatment. In Hock & J. Zubin (Eds.), *The evaluation of psychiatric treatment*. New York and London: Grune and Stratton, 1964. Killian, E. Effect of geriatric transfer on mortality rates. *Social Work*, January 1970, **15**(1), 19–26.

# 8

# The Posttransfer Fate of Relocated Patients

ELIZABETH W. MARKSON AND JOHN H. CUMMING

## Background

It is evident that the role of the state mental hospital is changing. Four developments in particular have contributed to the shift away from state hospital-centered care to community-based treatment. First, the proliferation of new psychotropic drugs has accelerated remission and permitted more rapid release of patients to the community.[1,2,3,4] Second, development of the notion of therapeutic milieu and therapeutic community has promoted the resocialization of patients and the redefining of staff roles. Third, and related to the redefining of the treatment environment, is the geographic decentralization of large state hospitals, a phenomenon eradicating or reducing reliance on custodial administrative patterns, thus promoting more rapid release of patients.

---

ELIZABETH W. MARKSON • Massachusetts Department of Mental Health, Boston, Massachusetts 02114.    JOHN H. CUMMING • Department of Health Services and Health Insurance, Victoria, British Columbia. The research reported herein was supported in part by NIMH grants No. MH-16498 and MH-20960 and by the New York State Department of Mental Hygiene. We should like to thank Isabel McCaffrey and Gary Levitz, both of whom proposed many of the ideas herein and assistance throughout the research. We should also like to thank Willard Van Horne for his help and Ralph Markson for preparation of the graphs. An earlier version of this paper was published in *The Gerontologist*, 1975.

And last, shifts in federal, state, and local funding modalities for treatment of the mentally ill have encouraged evolution of community-based facilities.[5]

These four interweaving skeins have produced a pattern of dramatically reduced inpatient censuses at state mental hospitals throughout the United States. From a high of nearly 600,000 in 1955, patients resident in state hospitals declined to 208,000 by 1971, and this trend has continued unabated to the present moment. Some outspoken critics of inpatient care, like Werner Mendel,[6,7] have suggested that all mental hospitals, public or private, should be dismantled, for the care provided therein is always expensive, always inefficient, frequently antitherapeutic, and never the treatment of choice. While the number of actual mental hospital closings is still very small, several states have considered or are considering closing mental hospitals, and most are reevaluating the function of these hospitals.

As a result of these changes, an acutely mentally ill person today is much less likely to be admitted as an inpatient to a state hospital than his counterpart ten years ago and if admitted, is less likely to stay for one or more months or to die while an inpatient. Yet most state hospitals still house a large number of chronic patients who, precisely because of their long careers as inpatients, are difficult to redirect to other facilities or to place in the community. The present study focuses on one such group of predominantly chronic patients during a period when their inpatient care was affected by massive budget reductions required by legislative action in New York State.

Almost every publicly supported system of services for the care of the mentally ill must suffer forced budget reductions from time to time. In New York in April 1971, the Division of Mental Health of the State Department of Mental Hygiene, faced with the necessity of reducing staff in order to cut costs, dismissed 1,167 state hospital employees. Most of the dismissals were limited to four institutions where there had been *less* than the average reduction in patient population; to compensate for the loss of staff at these four hospitals, 2,174 patients were transferred to other state hospitals serving the areas from which those patients had come or at which they could be more suitably served.

## The Study Group

Most of these 2,174 patients had been in a hospital for more than two years and were thus chronic patients; the mean length of hospitalization for the entire group was 19 years. The modal patient group (20%) had between 20 and 30 years of continuous hospital care, and 27% had been resident for 30 to 70 years. Seventy-one percent of the patients had a diagnosis of schizophrenia with chronic brain syndromes in second position. About 3 in 5 (57%) were women with a mean age of 57, and the remainder were men with a mean age of 53 years. The modal age group, comprising 29% of the 2,174 patients, was 60–69, and an additional 14% were 70 years of age or older at the time of transfer. In short, these 2,174 patients were for the most part older chronic schizophrenics. They were a group for whom discharge was not only statistically unlikely but who looked like poor release candidates from a clinical viewpoint. It was assumed that like Alice at the Mad Hatter's tea party, they must be mad or they would not be there.

Work by Aldrich and Mendkoff,[8] Blenkner,[9] and Markus, Blenkner, Bloom, and Downs[10] has suggested that the chronically disabled and the elderly face an excessively high risk of dying when they are transferred, even when the move seems to be an objective change for the better. The group of transfer patients who were 50 years of age or older thus seemed potentially at a high risk of dying as a response to their relocation. On the other hand, studies on the impact of mass patient transfer within a mental hospital suggest that transfer from one ward to another may be advantageous to chronic mental patients, especially to those "poorly adjusted" or regressed.[11,12,13] In short, the relocation of patients that occurred in response to the budget cuts presented a "natural experiment," a chance to explore the outcome of what in usual circumstances would not have happened—the forced relocation of a large group of lone-term, older chronic patients. The research reported here, utilizing sociodemographic data drawn from individual hospital and aftercare case records, focuses on the following questions:

1. Of the 2,174 patients relocated, was there a group who were more likely to die after the move than would be expected?
2. Of the surviving patients, was there a group released to the community within 90 days after transfer?
3. Was there a group of patients who were able to sustain themselves in the community?

## Results

### Mortality

To determine the impact of transfer upon patient mortality, the occurrence of deaths from date of transfer until approximately one year were examined. Only 3.9% of the 2,174 people tranferred had died as of

March 30, 1972 (an average of 313 days since transfer as patient relocation took place over a two-month period). Almost identical percentages
of men (3.9%) and women (4.0%) died, which probably reflects the fact
that the female patient group with a mean age of 57.5 was somewhat
older than the male group whose mean age was 53.9. Put differently,
men and women transferred were at an equal risk of death because the
women were slightly older.

For both sexes, death was related to age, those 65 years of age or
older being most likely to die. The mean age of geriatric patients ($N =$
494) transferred was 74.97, and ages ranged from 65 to 95. Slightly less
than one in ten of the elderly transfer patients died during the eleven
month period following their relocation.

A useful comparison of mortality of the 494 transferred elderly
patients may be made to two relatively small control groups of geriatric
patients, selected for contrast because they, like the transfer patients,
were ambulatory and relatively physically healthy but were not transferred. One group consisted of 140 chronic inpatients on the geriatric
wards of two mental hospitals, and the other was composed of 35 old
people living in the community and attending a psychogeriatric day
care center. Transfer patients, inpatients, and day care patients all had a
mean age between 74 and 75. About 6% of the patients attending day
care and about 9% of those at the two state hospitals died within an
eleven-month period, as compared to 9% of the transferred old people
during the same time period; there is no statistically significant difference among these rates.

That there are no striking differences in the death rates among
these three sets of relatively healthy elderly strengthens the observation
of previous investigators[10,14,15,16,17,18] that the excessive mortality
reported in a number of relocation studies may be a reflection not of
moving but of specific patient characteristics. These include poor physical health, and mental confusion, themselves often prodromal signs of
death. Put another way, relocation may hasten an already impending
death but does not necessarily speed mortality among the relatively
well.

## Who Was Released?

The hospitals from which the patients came had the reputation of
providing humane and conservative care. They had, however, been
reducing their population at a slower rate than other hospitals in the
state, and one of the purposes of the move, given the necessity of
making it, was to place patients in more active hospitals and improve

their chance of discharge. Further, it has been widely reported that overcrowding—or as it has been euphemistically called, "statistical pressure"—tends to accelerate the rate of discharge from a hospital or a ward. That is, there are definite norms in any ward, subscribed to by patients and staff about the appropriate number and types of patients in that ward. Changes in the type or number of patients in a given ward may cause as much or more anxiety among the staff as among patients. For example, shifts in admission or discharge rates may, as some investigators have suggested,[3,19,20] disrupt the balance of the social system of the ward and require role reallocation or the development of new norms before the system is in balance again. There are definite if unspoken hospital or ward preconceptions about the "right" number or range of types of patients. When either of these is disrupted, the ward supervisor and staff feel vaguely uncomfortable and attempt to transfer to other wards patients who "don't fit" numerically or socially. If this effort fails, the staff begins to inspect patient groups for the most likely candidates for discharge even in wards where discharge hitherto has been unknown.[19,21] This process is not as mechanistic as it first sounds; the staff probably selects potential candidates for release by beginning to treat certain patients as if they were "normal" and finding out how they respond. Thus expectations change, and since "ego's expectations are alter's sanctions," patients start to act "normally" and are declared suitable for discharge.

This analysis focuses on patients discharged during the first 90 days after transfer. In total, 375, or a little over 17% of the 2,174 patients transferred, were discharged within 90 days from the 13 hospitals receiving them. Given the overcrowding argument just outlined, one might expect releases to be fairly evenly distributed among the various hospitals, but rates of release varied considerably, from zero at one institution to 88% at another. The hospitals may be divided into three groups. The first group of three hospitals had a high discharge rate and released 75.6% of the 271 patients received within 90 days. The second group of four hospitals had a moderate discharge rate; they released 12.9% of the 1,245 patients they received. The third group, consisting of six hospitals with a low rate of discharge, released only 1.5% of the 658 patients they had received. Hospital policy thus seems a significant variable in accounting for the differences in release rates among the three groups.

*Factors in Release—Demographic Characteristics.* To test the hypothesis that hospital policy was the decisive factor in determining release of the patients transferred rather than some attributes of the patients themselves, we examined a series of characteristics of the transfer

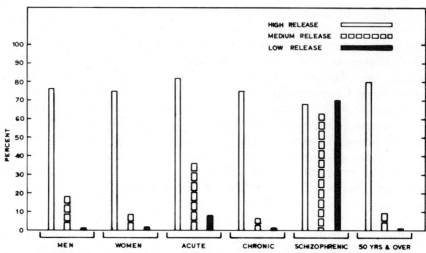

Figure 1. Proportion of transferred patients released within 90 days of those received, by hospital discharge group.

patients (see Figure 1). Although, as one might expect, patients with less than two years of hospitalization were generally and significantly more likely to be released than their chronic counterparts, there was considerable variation among hospitals in this pattern. The high discharge hospitals released 75.1% of the patients with two or more years of continuous hospitalization while the hospitals in the medium group released only 6.6% of their chronic patients, and in the low group, only 1.5% of the chronic patients received in the transfer had been released within the 90-day period.

It might have been that the age of patients explained some of the variation observed among the hospitals. Older patients, regardless of their chronicity, are notoriously difficult to place in the community. This was not always the case, however, as high discharge hospitals released 4 in 5 of its patients 50 years of age and older as compared to the moderate release group, which let go slightly less than 1 in 10, and to the low group, releasing less than 2 in 100.

Nor was the sex of the patient a significant variable in accounting for the differences in discharge rates among hospitals; at the high release institutions, about 3 in 4 male *or* female patients were released to the community. At the low release hospitals, slightly more than 1 in 100 men or women were released.

*Diagnosis.* Nor were the patients released from the various hospitals drastically dissimilar with respect to diagnosis. As stated earlier,

71% of the patients in the transfer were schizophrenic; 66%, 67%, and 79% of the people sent to the high, medium, and low discharge hospitals, respectively, were schizophrenic. In general, the diagnosis of released patients was a reflection of this; in most of the hospitals, remarkably similar proportions of schizophrenics to the proportions received in transfer were discharged. There seems no evidence to show that any difference in diagnosis of patients received at the various hospitals accounted for the differential rates of release.

*Placement.* It seems, then, that whether one is likely to be released or not is dependent on some aspect of hospital policy other than patient characteristics or overcrowding. One significant indicator of hospital policy affecting release is the type of placement made for patients sent back to the community (see Figure 2). The high discharge group of hospitals placed 71% of the patients they released within 90 days in a congregate care facility, such as an old age home, a nursing home, or an adult home, where supervision was provided. Only about 7% of the patients released from the moderate discharge group of hospitals and 10% of those from the low group were placed in such facilities; the preference in these two sets of hospitals was clearly for placement in one's own home, with relatives, or in so-called single-room-occupancy

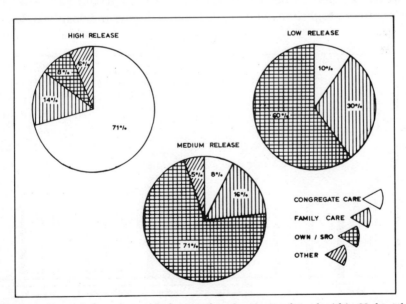

Figure 2. Type of placement made for transferred patients released within 90 days, by hospital discharge group.

dwellings where little if any supervision was provided. Put another way, patients released from the high discharge group of hospitals apparently were not required to be as fully self-sufficient before leaving the hospital as were those, from moderate and low release hospitals, who were sent to presumably less protected settings. That such large proportions of chronic patients 50 years of age or older who had few close ties with the world outside the hospital were sent out by the high release hospitals is, in large part, a reflection of the readiness of this group of facilities to use "low risk" congregate care facilities. Hospitals using fewer congregate care placements apparently discharged primarily only those patients that were felt to be good "community risks."

## "Success" in the Community

Of course not all those who were released, whether to the more supervised environs of a congregate care facility or to the less supervised settings of their own homes or boarding houses, made a stable adjustment in the community, at least on the first attempt (see Figure 3). During the period of postrelease follow-up (an average of 313 days from the time of transfer), 39% of those released within 90 days after transfer had returned to the hospital. Stringency of release procedures was not, however, a factor in determining which patients would be returned. Very similar proportions of patients failed, whether the hospital releas-

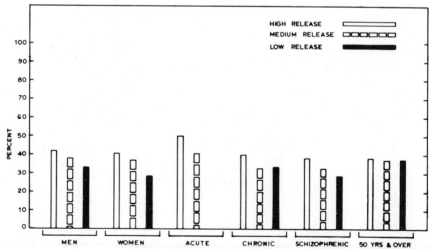

Figure 3. Proportion of released transfer patients who failed in the community of those released, by hospital discharge group.

ing them was a high, medium, or low release facility. In sum, whether strict or lenient criteria were used to screen patients for release made no difference in terms of community tenure. Nor did age, sex, diagnosis, or type of community placement relate to tenure in the community during the follow-up period. The likelihood of return to the hospital was, however, significantly linked to role complaints about patients' inability to care for themselves or to do what was expected in the community setting. Eighty-four percent of those about whom such a complaint was made returned to the hospital as compared to only 2% of those not returned but about whom a role complaint was made ($\chi^2 = 30.099$, $df = 1$, $p < .001$). That actual performance in the community was perhaps the best indicator of success or failure in the setting is given further support when the scores on a role index which included employment, self-care, and role failure of those staying in the community are compared to the scores of those returning. Those patients returning to the hospital had a mean score of 5.26 ( a perfect score = 9.0). People who stayed in the community throughout the study period had a somewhat higher score of 6.05; this difference is statistically significant ($t = 5.015$, $p < .001$).

Despite the different discharge and release patterns among the thirteen hospitals that received transfer patients, once the patients are themselves released there is suprisingly little difference in community tenure. Although relatively "bad risk" patients were released in abundance to congregate care facilities, they did no worse than their more highly selected counterparts from the more conservative hospitals with lower release rates. In large part, the variation between hospitals in the three different release groups can be explained by the experience of each hospital in "running down" its population. That is, those hospitals generally ranking *high* in decreasing their census were more likely to release a large proportion of their transfer patients within 90 days than were those hospitals ranking low on rundown ($\rho = .82$). Put differently, hospitals releasing transfer patients with the greatest alacrity were aiso extremely efficient in running down their census. Norms of overcrowding appear to be applied in varying degrees, each institution adapting to additional patients in keeping with both its overall treatment philosophy and commonly held staff cutoff points regarding what is mental illness requiring hospitalization and what constitutes a satisfactory placement outside the hospital. It would seem that, given ward overcrowding, one must be observably "crazier" to stay as a patient in a hospital such as the three in the high discharge category than to stay that same period in a hospital in the low release group of hospitals.

## Discussion

What then may be learned from the experience of the transfer patients? First, while the literature has suggested that to the chronic patients any move may be interpreted as threatening and involving painful readjustment, we could find no evidence that forced relocation of a group of relatively physically healthy, chronic, predominantly schizophrenic patients from one institution to another is sufficiently stressful to cause a higher than normal death rate among them. Nor were elderly patients at any apparent high risk of dying when relocated; their mortality did not differ from that of two other relatively physically healthy groups of geriatric patients—one served in the community, the other in state hospital—not relocated during a similar time period.

Second, it is clear that a sizable number of patients of all ages can live outside a mental hospital, even though the setting in which many are placed is congregate care. Ideally, perhaps, each patient would be discharged to less institutional settings than were those from the high release hospitals. What is apparent, however, is that these chronic patients did not require *mental* hospitalization, although it is not certain whether the long history of institutionalization of these patients might not have rendered them incapable of totally independent living.

Third, it seems evident that the norms and practices of the mental hospital are more significant in determining whether a patient is released or retained than his mental condition. Specifically, the patient rundown experience of a hospital seems the most crucial factor in determining whether or not a given patient will be released. Small, relatively new acute facilities, such as the hospitals in the high release group, are especially likely to use community facilities for the placement of chronic patients.

Fourth, neither the chronicity of the patient nor his diagnosis was particularly important in determining whether or not he succeeded in remaining in the community. Rather, his physical health and social role competency were the decisive factors.

In short, New York's experience with the forced relocation of primarily chronic and older mental patients suggests that a large proportion of these patients can be efficaciously rechanneled into community-based facilities. But, given that this pattern of care is possible, is it desirable? In our research, we found little evidence to suggest that concerted attention was being given to the quality of life, the rehabilitation, and increased social competency of patients discharged to the community. This would have required a different and more expensive organization of posthospital care than the department had available, nor did most individual community facilities possess these resources. On the one hand, there is growing evidence that the chronic mental patient "shuffles to oblivion" when released to the community.[22,23] Yet, at the same time, it has been well documented over the years that the chronic mental hospital ward is no satisfactory substitute for community living.

Since 1971, as growing numbers of patients have been released from mental hospitals not only in New York State but elsewhere, the need for effective aftercare programs to prevent shuffles to oblivion has been stressed. Indeed, it seems clear that, if chronic patients are to remain in the community successfully, they may require aggressive outreach services to provide continual medication, emotional supports, and rehabilitation, and to ensure quality of life. Whether aftercare, however, is in fact either available or the treatment of choice for most patients returned to the community remains moot. While some studies have indicated that ex-patients receiving follow-up at a clinic experienced significantly lower rates of rehospitalization than their controls who received none,[24,25] there is also opposing evidence suggesting that ex-patients attending an aftercare clinic are more likely to be readmitted to hospital than those not attending aftercare.[26,27]

Perhaps at least part of the difficulty in assessing the impact of aftercare in preventing rehospitalization or enhancing quality of life is due to a lack of uniformity in program standards and in services. Some aftercare programs are mediocre and do not provide comprehensive care based upon a rational prescription according to patient needs. Also, because community-based alternatives to continued inpatient care are relatively new (and sometimes expensive), aftercare services may be focused more on counseling, psychotherapy, and medication than on needed social services such as vocational training, financial assistance, resocialization, and housing. In a recent Massachusetts survey of 88 randomly selected adult patients, released during a 7-month period during 1974 to the community (excluding congregate care facilities), for example, 85% were referred for aftercare. Only 1 in 5 of these referred received help on environmental problems such as housing, financial support, or employment, while 4 in 5 received counseling, supportive therapy, or medication.[28] It seems likely that a greater proportion of these patients could have benefited from a more pragmatic approach to their environmental problems than they were offered.

A second problem in delivering aftercare is the absence of continuity of care in some locales. Too often, no organized system of aftercare may exist in a given catchment area. Put another way, state hospital staff may, for a variety of reasons including financial, define aftercare as a community responsibility; the community in turn defines it as a hospital responsibility and no specific contracts for provision of service or demarkation of responsibility for ex-patients are in force.

Furthermore, often there is no administrative mechanism to ascertain whether those people referred for aftercare actually receive the recommended services. It would be valuable to know not only whether an aftercare plan has been implemented but also the extent to which the plan could not be completed and the reasons therefor. With such data, a mental health system may evaluate its services, plan for new ones as needed, and reallocate fiscal resources to develop viable community-based alternatives.

## References

1. Cole, J. D., & Gerard, R. W. (Eds.). *Psychopharmacology: Problems in evaluation.* Washington, D.C.: National Academy of Sciences, 1959.
2. Pasamanick, B., Scarpitti, F. R., & Dinitz, S. *Schizophrenics in the community.* New York: Appleton-Century-Crofts, 1967.
3. Cumming, J., & Cumming, E. Social equilibrium and social change in the large mental hospital. In M. Greenblatt, D. S. Levison, & R. H. Williams (Eds.), *The patient and the mental hospital.* Glencoe, Illinois: Free Press, 1957.
4. Jones, M. S. *Social psychiatry in practice: The idea of a therapeutic community.* Baltimore: Penguin Books, 1968.
5. Bloom, B. L. *Community mental health: A historical and critical analysis.* Morristown, New Jersey: General Learning Corporation, 1973.
6. Mendel, W., Rapport, S., & Glasser, J. *High quality, low cost prepaid psychiatric service.* Paper presented at the American Psychiatric Association, Hawaii, 1973.
7. Mendel, W. Dismantling the mental hospital. In *Where is my home: Proceedings of a Conference on the Closing of State Mental Hospitals.* Menlo Park, California: Stanford Research Institute, 1974.
8. Aldrich, C., & Mendkoff, E. Relocation of the aged and disabled: A mortality study. *Journal of the American Geriatric Society,* 1963, III.
9. Blenkner, M. Environment change and the aging individual. *The Gerontologist,* 1967, **7**.
10. Markus, E., Blenkner, M., Bloom, M., & Downs, T. Relocation stress and the aged. In H. T. Blumenthal (Ed.), *Interdisciplinary topics in gerontology* (Vol. 7). Basel: S. Karger, 1970, pp. 60–71.
11. Greenblatt, M., Landy, D., Hyde, R., & Bockoven, J. S. Rehabilitation of the mentally ill: Impact of a project upon hospital structure. *American Journal of Psychiatry,* 1958, **114**, 986–992.
12. Bloch, F., Barrington, L., Burke, J., & Lafave, H. Changes in mental hospital programs as seen by patients and ward personnel. *Diseases of the Nervous System,* 1964, **25**, 601–610.
13. Zlotowski, M., & Cohen, D. Effects of the environmental change upon behavior of hospitalized schizophrenic patients. *Journal of Clinical Psychology,* 1968, **24**, 470–475.

14. Killian, E. C. Effects of geriatric transfer on mortality rates. *Social Work*, 1970, **15**, 19–26.
15. Lawton, M. P., & Nahemow, L. Ecology and the aging process. In C. Esdorfer & M. P. Lawton (Eds.), *The psychology of adult development and aging*. Washington, D.C.: American Psychological Association, 1973.
16. Markson, E. W. The geriatric house of death. *Aging and Human Development*, 1970, **1**, 37–49.
17. Markson, E. W., Kwoh, A., Cumming, J., & Cumming, E. Alternatives to hospitalization for psychiatrically ill geriatric patients. *American Journal of Psychiatry*, 1971, **127**, 1055–1062.
18. Shahinian, S., Goldfarb, A., & Turner, H. *Death rate in relocated residents of nursing homes*. Presented at the annual meeting of the Gerontological Society, New York, November 1966.
19. Kraus, P. Ward assignments and patient movement in a large psychiatric hospital. In M. Greenblatt, D. S. Levinson, & R. H. Williams (Eds.), *The patient and the mental hospital*. Glencoe, Illinois: Free Press, 1957.
20. Lafave, G. Reducing admissions and increasing discharges. *Canada's Mental Health*, 1966, **14**, 7–11.
21. Ullman, L. *Institution and outcome*. New York: Pergamon Press, 1967.
22. Reich, R., & Siegal, L. Psychiatry under siege: The chronically mentally ill shuffle to oblivion. *Psychiatric Annals*, 1973, **3** (November).
23. British Medical Journal. *Rootless wanderers* (editorial). July 7, 1973.
24. Orlinsky, N., & D'Elia, E. Rehospitalization of the schizophrenic patient. *Archives of General Psychiatry*, 1964, **10**, 47–54.
25. Purvis, S. A., and Miskimins, R. W. Effects of community follow-up on posthospital adjustment of psychiatric patients. *Community Mental Health Journal*, 1970, **6**, 374–82.
26. Herjanic, M. Does it pay to discharge the chronic patient? *Acta Psychiatrica Scandinavica*, 1969, **45**, 53–61.
27. Penick, S. B. Short-term acute psychiatric care: A follow-up study. *American Journal of Psychiatry*, 1971, **38**, 1626–30.
28. Van Horne, W. Personal communication, 1975.

# 9

# Community-Based Sheltered Care

## STEVEN P. SEGAL AND URI AVIRAM

In the past twelve years a new and largely ungoverned system of community-based sheltered care for the ex-mental patient has evolved in California. The evolution of this privately owned residential care system is a major unanticipated consequence of a national trend toward community care for the mentally ill initiated by the 1963 Community Mental Health Centers Act. While the participants in the Joint Commission on Mental Illness and Health conceived of multiple aftercare services, they did not foresee the development of privately owned, sheltered-care facilities on an ad hoc basis as a primary posthospital resource.[1] Because of the ad hoc nature of this system, there are numerous unanswered questions concerning its origin, its character, and its impact, both on the individual and on the community.

In California, the impetus for the development of this residential care system is found in two state government policies. The first was initiated in the 1963 California Welfare regulations which made financial support available to persons disabled by mental illness under the Categorical Aid to the Disabled Program.[2] The availability of financial resources under the 1963 ATD regulations provided an alternative to hospital life. This was particularly true for the proportion of mental

STEVEN P. SEGAL • School of Social Welfare, University of California, Berkeley, California 94720. URI AVIRAM • Tel Aviv University, Tel Aviv, Israel.

patients who remained institutionalized for no other reason than their lack of finances and inability to obtain immediate employment.

The second policy, formalized in the Short-Doyle Act of 1958 and the Lanterman-Petris-Short Act of 1968, has fostered the growth of the residential care system by significantly reducing the use of state hospitals. The Lanterman-Petris-Short Act accomplished this through its provisions which make involuntary detention of the mentally ill for any long period of time extremely difficult. The Short-Doyle legislation achieved this goal through financial inducements to counties for reducing their use of 24-hour inpatient care.[3]

In the summer of 1972, after a series of media exposés on the living conditions of sheltered-care residents and on a tragic fire in which several residents were killed, the state passed a licensing bill (Brathwaite, AB 344) to regulate residential services offered to the 18–65-year-old socially dependent group—such regulations had previously existed only for children and the aged. Given the mandate to establish guidelines for facilities offering adult residential services, the state was, for the first time, confronted with the need to gain some understanding of how these organizations operated as aftercare settings. Until this time no such knowledge existed because in most areas of the state all that had been needed to open such a facility was a business license. Thus, our project team received state funds to do a study of community-based sheltered care for the mentally ill.

## Studying Community-Based Sheltered Care

Our project team consisting of two research social workers and three doctoral research assistants received support from the California State Department of Health in October 1972, to begin to develop a factual basis for understanding the service system. In order to further our knowledge of the sheltered-care situation, our team gathered information on its political and social dynamics through open-ended interviews and observation. During this phase of our study, we contacted 134 people—including former mental patients living in sheltered care, social workers, political decision makers, operators of residential care facilities, CCMHC administrators, and others. In the second phase of the study, we completed a survey of a probability sample of residents and operators which was geared to provide precise information on the characteristics of these groups in California and to answer several questions concerning the nature of the sheltered-care environment as an aftercare setting. In the survey phase of the study, we initiated structured interviews with 234 facility operators and 499 residents, a representative sample of all nonretarded former mental hospital patients between the ages of 18 and 65 living in sheltered care.

Considering sheltered care as an aftercare setting in this preliminary report on our findings, the two questions which seem most important to address are (1) whether life in this type of facility and in the state hospital community differ significantly or tend to have similar consequences for resident functioning; (2) what is the potential of the sheltered-care system as an aftercare environment for the released mental hospital patient in the current political and social context. Before we can address these two important questions, however, it seems necessary to consider an even more basic one—i.e., what is the current nature of sheltered care?

## The Sheltered-Care Environment

The cumulative effect of the 1963 ATD, Lanterman-Petris-Short, and Short-Doyle regulations was to foster a proliferation of sheltered-care facilities. These facilities developed in part as a response to the creation of a "voucher" system—though not so named—which enabled members of socially dependent groups to purchase supervised residential care through specially designated ATD grants. Upon the resident's leaving a supervised residential care environment, the value of the ATD check is substantially reduced. Thus, in effect, the ATD check is a voucher for this type of care. The voucher system model has a built-in assumption of consumer control. Sheltered-care operators, however, have managed to maintain a high degree of control over their residents, thus creating a stable and dependent group of consumers. The lack of control the former mental patient population has over these vouchers is illustrated in the report of 52.5% of the residents that the checks come to the operator who opens the mail and has his boarder sign the full amount over to him. The operator later returns a small proportion of this money to the resident for his own personal needs (currently $33 from a $283-a-month grant). In 16.7% of the cases, a conservator was involved in the payment of the rent. Only about one out of four residents receive their mail unopened and pay the operator themselves. These common practices dispel even the illusion of consumer control.

The second factor influencing the growth of sheltered care was the release of large groups of individuals from state hospitals under the California mental health acts. These regulations provided the new facility operator with a stable and largely dependent resident population without any requirement to meet quality of care standards. This created a business opportunity for the small entrepreneur to provide residential care to the mentally ill, and it seems to have opened up a new avenue of upward social mobility for attendants, nurses, aides, and other former service personnel who wished to go into business. It enabled the family wanting to make some extra money on the side to open their home to the mentally ill and provided a new market for already established providers of residential services, e.g., owners of boarding homes catering to students in university areas or owners of old hotels catering to an aged or largely transient population. One employee of a Long Beach, New York, sheltered-care facility who began working as a payroll clerk at the hotel when it served wealthy New Yorkers on summer holidays said that she was pleased with the hotel's transformation because "if we had not taken this step, we would have had to close for lack of business."[4] All these types of facilities joined the small number of professionally operated halfway houses and professionally certified family care homes to constitute the large number of residential care units currently providing services to the mentally ill in local communities.

Obviously, then, life in board and care is not a uniform experience but varies considerably. Imagine yourself in the position of a recently released mental patient. If you are fortunate enough to have a social worker who actually takes you around to three facilities prior to choosing your residence, you might be faced with three totally different potential life experiences. (In Los Angeles, as in other areas of the state, prospective residents are supposed to be given a choice of one of the next three facilities which come up on a rotating list.) You might find facilities which varied in size from one to 300 people. You might observe a facility that functioned like a boarding house or one that was run like a minihospital. You could come across a place which looked very much like a flophouse or one which looked like a resort. You could find a home, a commune, or a therapeutic community. Any combination along these differing dimensions and several others are available to a greater or lesser degree under the rubric of sheltered care.

The growth of the sheltered-care system has been rapid. Morrissey notes that there were only 13,000 individuals in family-care placement in the United States in 1964.[5] In 1969, using a definition of the halfway house which would encompass most residential home-care placements, Glasscote and colleagues note the existence of only 148 such facilities, with a total bed capacity of 2,507 for mentally ill residents.[6] These figures, when compared to our summer, 1973, census estimate of 12,400 nonretarded former hospital patients between 18 and 65 years of age in California sheltered-care facilities, demonstrate the rapid development of this aftercare facility system.[7]

Given the rapid, unplanned growth and the diversity of the sheltered-care system, how has it dealt with the negative consequences
fostered by its predecessor—the state hospital?

## Sheltered Care and the Negative Consequences of the State Hospital

The negative consequences of hospitalization can be attributed to
three factors: extended hospitalization, degree of confinement, and a
desocializing environment. Looking first at duration of hospitalization,
Kramer found that the chance of a patient ever leaving a mental hospital
after one year of continuous residence approaches zero.[8] The consequences of long-term hospitalization have been described by Russell
Barton and John Wing in the concept of "institutional neurosis," that is,
dependence of the individual on his institutional environment.[9] External social roles break down and the patient's place in society is lost.
Institutional neurosis, as observed by Wing, does not necessarily
involve bizarre symptomatology.

The degree of confinement seems to have the most detrimental
effects on people in relation to bizarre symptomatology. This is evident
in the miraculous cures reported by Pinel in the opening up of two Paris
asylums in 1792 and is continually rediscovered by individuals responsible for the care of the mentally ill. In the early 1950s, prior to the
introduction of psychoactive drugs, Dr. T. P. Rees initiated the mod-
ern-day open-hospital movement in England.[10] Rees's concept of the
open hospital did not involve extensive release of patients to the
community, but simply the unlocking of wards. This change in itself
significantly reduced the amount of bizarre, asocial behavior exhibited
in these hospitals.

These findings relating to "institutional neurosis" and bizarre
symptomatology are consistent with the approach of French psychiatrist, Henri Ellenberger, which compares a state mental hospital with a
zoological park. Ellenberger points out with respect to confinement that
animals in zoos are likely to experience the "trauma of captivity,"
including prolonged stupor, hunger strikes, severe agitation, and the
manifestation of violent symptoms. He also reports the phenomenon of
"nestling" among animals in zoos whereby they take root in their
environment after being there for a good deal of time.[11] This type of
behavior is consistent with Wing's findings on institutionalization
which note that the key factor in creating this phenomenon is time
itself.[12]

The works of Erving Goffman and Jack Zussman have illuminated
the third factor in the negative impact of hospitalization.[13] They
emphasize the necessity of the patient's continuing to be perceived as

an individual in his own right if his social responses to others are not to deteriorate. Ernest Gruenberg has appropriately termed this deterioration the *social breakdown syndrome,* thereby stressing the importance of the patient's continuing to conduct himself as a human being. In the past, institutions have taken the symbols of individuality away from patients: their own clothing, grooming utensils, a place to keep personal items with which to prepare to face the everyday world (one expects to have his clothes in his bedroom rather than having them stored in a separate section of the building that can only be reached through common areas).

In considering the influence of duration of stay in a sheltered-care facility, our data indicate that 55% of the population thought that it would be at least "all right" to stay in their current living arrangement for a long period of time. It thus seems that a similar type of settling in to one's current environment observed among long-term hospital patients is characteristic of the response of the sheltered-care population. However, it might be hypothesized—given the duration of many unhappy marriages and Ellenberger's observations on "nestling behavior" in animals in zoos—that we are in fact observing in Wing's concept of institutionalization a more general pattern of human response to a stable situation as opposed to the specific reaction of a mental patient becoming dependent on the hospital environment.

Confinement in the gross sense of the term and depriving the individual of the basic symbols of individuality have been ensured against in California's proposed licensing regulations. In guarding against these two factors, the ability to monitor system abuses will be extremely important.

To examine the issue of confinement: Residents were asked what was the *most* important difference between their life in the hospital and their life in sheltered care; 53.3% indicated that the major difference was that they were "free to come and go." The next most frequent response also emphasized personal freedom; 14.4% said it was that they were "free to plan their own activities." Whereas all other categories had a low positive response, 8.6% did choose the category "not very much difference."

It thus appears that at least with respect to confinement, the negative consequences of hospitalization will not be repeated on a broad scale.

Although residents in sheltered care universally wear their own clothes, not uniforms, the protection of the resident's right to symbols of individuality is crucial, especially in the larger facilities—some of which approach the size and character of a small chronic hospital. In addition, and perhaps the most important finding in our study, is the significant positive relationship between becoming involved within the sheltered-care facility and reaching out independently toward involvement in the outside community. To the extent that the sheltered-care facility environment promotes internal involvement, it will promote outreach among its residents and avoid duplication of the desocializing aspects of the "back ward" of the state hospital.

Given the social character of the sheltered-care environment, its de-emphasis of confinement, and the possibility that the observed pattern of residents settling into their current living situation is characteristic of any social group in a stable setting, it seems that many of the negative consequences of the state hospital have indeed been avoided in sheltered care. Thus, our second study question—what is the potential of the sheltered-care system as an aftercare environment in its current political and social context—is the critical one.

## Political–Social Dynamics of the Sheltered-Care System

The rapid growth of sheltered care in California has had two major social and political results which have substantially influenced the character of this system as an aftercare setting.

First, it precipitated a considerable fear response from local communities, and second, it led to the development of distinct politically active interest groups whose concerns centered on sheltered care.

*Social Exclusion of the Sheltered-Care Resident.* The fear response to what the *San Jose Mercury* (November 16, 1971) called a "mass invasion of mental patients" has made sheltered care a community-wide issue throughout California.

Previous studies of public attitudes toward the mentally ill have indicated that the inability to explain a person's actions in some reasonable way and in the context of one's own life experience is key in interpreting behavior as mentally disordered. The public sees the behavior of the mentally ill as unpredictable and therefore posing a personal threat. The "raving maniac" is what comes to mind when most people talk of the mentally ill.[14]

Perhaps the best illustration of the reaction to eliminating state hospitals as means of removing the mentally ill from the local community is the recent development of alternative measures to keep the sheltered-care home out of local areas. These measures directed against sheltered-care facilities include the use of zoning ordinances, city ordinances, and regulations especially relating to fire safety. They also include informal mechanisms such as neighborhood pressure and bureaucratic maneuvering.

One example of these types of actions is a city's demand that every

new sheltered-care home operator obtain a permit from the fire marshal. A week later the city announced a moratorium, suspending the
authority of the fire marshal to issue permits for a specified period of
time which was later extended. Thus those who operated homes for the
mentally ill in the community did not have enough time to get the
required permits nor could anyone start a new facility operation in that
community.[15]

It is our impression that the influence of these exclusionary tactics
is not a minor one. It was apparent that during the year prior to the
study, many new facilities opened and many also closed. Approximately 19% of our sample of 214 operators have received complaints
from their neighbors. Fourteen percent have had complaints about their
facilities made to the local authorities, and 4% of the interviewed
operators indicated that they have been threatened or harassed by
neighbors.

Contrary to the popular myth which states that complaints occur
only at the time the facility opens and that afterwards the neighborhood
will adapt to the presence of the mentally ill, our findings indicate that
80% of the complaints made to the operator and 68% of the complaints
made about the facilities to authorities are made after the facility has
been opened "awhile." These facts do not rule out the ultimate adaptation of the community to the mentally ill, but they do indicate that this
adaptation may be a long and arduous process.

Homeowners' groups in the most well-to-do sections of Los Angeles have been most vocal in their efforts to keep sheltered-care homes
out of the single-family residential zone. They have not had a sheltered-
care facility in their neighborhood and most likely never will. It therefore seems that their opposition is based on fear stemming from the
public's stereotype of the mentally ill.

In addressing the question of a community fear reaction, one must
ask about the validity of the public's stereotype regarding the mentally
ill and whether it is applicable to those individuals living in sheltered-
care homes.

Stereotypes do not exist in a vacuum. They usually have some basis
in fact, though these facts may be wrongly perceived. Miller reports that
approximately 9% of her ex-patient cohort in the San Francisco Bay
Area were released to a sheltered-living environment. Those released to
sheltered-care situations were, and traditionally have been, older, long-
term hospital patients, rather than the younger and perhaps more
transient group.[16] The evidence comparing violent crime in the released
hospital population with violent crime in the general population is
equivocal. Although a recent study in California found higher convic-

tion rates in the total released patient population than in the general population,[17] previous reports have indicated little difference between the two groups, or a lower rate in the released patient group.[18] One finding, however, consistent in all these studies, is that the older people in both groups have the lowest rates of violent crime. These studies are of the total released patient group. The extent to which they are representative of the small proportion of released patients who go to sheltered care is not certain.

The initial findings of our study relating to this question involve facility operators' reports about their residents. We asked operators if any of their residents had been picked up by the police in the past year and the reasons for these police contacts. Forty percent of the operators indicated that at least one of their residents had been picked up by the police in the past year. Yet only one operator of the 92 operators who answered the question affirmatively said that the reason for being picked up by the police was the commission of a violent act. This single violent act involved an arrest on charges of armed robbery. Only 4% of the police contacts involved bizarre behavior. The most frequent reason given for having a resident picked up by the police—40% of the affirmative responses—involved a resident "lost and wandering around the neighborhood." Whether this happened because the resident was actually lost or because a neighbor, worrying about the resident standing in front of the house, requested the pickup is unknown. The nature of these statistics, however, should lead to an appreciation of the vulnerability of this group, not its dangerousness. It would seem that the group of released patients going to residential care are feared more for their supposed potential danger than for their actual threat to the public.

*The Political Climate of Sheltered Care.* The second result of the rapid growth of residential care facilities in California was the development of distinct, politically active interest groups whose concerns center on sheltered care. The concern of these interest groups for the needs of the sheltered-care population is perhaps best illustrated by their agreement that "quality of care" is the most important issue to be considered. This is a goal acceptable to all factions, although each faction has defined resident need in terms of their own interests or at least their own perceptions of the problem.

If we take the Los Angeles situation as an example, the homeowners' groups have defined quality of care in terms of supervision and medical services. Speaking rather derisively about "mama–papa operations," they emphatically point out that only a large facility is capable of providing proper care. This perception of quality of care has brought them into an uneasy alliance with the operators of large sheltered-care facilities which are not located in single-family residential zones. This definition of quality of care is consistent with their stated desire to exclude sheltered care from single-family residential areas.

The mental health professionals have defined quality of care largely in terms of the delivery of services. Such a definition, needless to say, accords mental health professionals a principal role in the field. The professional group has argued for more open zoning, supporting the benefit of the small, "home type" environment under professional supervision as a key factor in providing high-quality care. Such a facility, it was noted by one administrator, is the most amenable to professional control and sanctions. Mental health professionals also support the halfway house concept when it is sponsored by the professional community and imbued with a liberal dose of psychiatric ideology. An interesting consequence of this conception is that several more market-minded sheltered-care operators have learned psychiatric jargon and the "right" answers. A few have hired public relations people to translate their efforts in the most appropriate professional language. I do not mean to imply that these alternatives would not provide a responsible and high-quality system. It should be pointed out, however, that a professionally controlled system may have some drawbacks if resident independence is a primary and realistic goal. Moving out from the protective umbrella of the mental health profession, in this situation, may be a necessary step toward independence.

The sheltered-care operators have accepted a definition of quality of care in terms of their own self-betterment—becoming better care givers through training. Such a system is congruent with their need for accreditation and legitimacy in what is now, in several areas of California, a highly competitive market. The provision of training and legitimacy to the operator group seems to be a good means of upgrading care. A recent report issued by the State Department of Health emphasized the fact that the more trained operators were less likely to have received "inadequate" ratings by survey interviewers in providing needed services to their residents.[19] In training and licensing operators, however, we may be creating a new professional cadre and, in fact, may be simply extending the principles and prejudices of hospital care into the community—thus losing the benefits of the more natural, though perhaps not as elegant, environment.

Finally, a consumer-oriented group of sheltered-care residents has defined quality of care in terms of the guarantees of resident civil rights. More particularly, it argues the right of the resident not to be excluded from community resources open to the general public simply on the basis of his ex-patient status.

These conceptions of quality of care all have great merit and potential, yet they are by no means congruent. The interests embodied in them and the community fear reaction discussed earlier have come to the forefront in zoning controversies that have erupted throughout California. An example of a zoning controversy over sheltered care clearly illustrates the conflict of personal interest embodied in these quality-of-care conceptions.

Consider the controversy in Los Angeles county during the past three years. Different proposals regarding zoning ordinances would have restricted sheltered-care facilities in certain zones and limited their development in others. Homeowners and operators considered a compromise which would have meant the end of future facilities in single-family residential zones. This action obviously would have discouraged the future development of small facilities.

Another solution in Los Angeles would have permitted small facilities in single-family residential zones, while drastically limiting the zones in which larger facilities were permitted. This solution threatened the existence of currently operating larger facilities in more residential type areas and would have placed significant limits on the types of neighborhoods in which these facilities could operate.

All of the proposed compromises considered in the county were *more* restrictive than state legislation, which allows a home with up to six individuals to operate in a single-family residential zone. Thus, all the proposed compromises would have placed more extensive restrictions on the civil rights of sheltered-care residents than currently specified in state law.

Finally, operators of sheltered-care homes seemed primarily interested in ensuring their continued existence without regard to future facilities. This, perhaps, is the end that has been achieved by virtue of the current limbo in which the system finds itself due to the failure of the Los Angeles City Council to adopt a compromise.

## The Potential of Sheltered Care

In the context of social exclusion and well-motivated yet vested-interest politics, what is the potential of the sheltered-care system as an aftercare environment for the released mental hospital patient?

The development of the sheltered-care environment as a system of aftercare for the chronic mental patient represents the first major change in providing residential service to this population in at least 100 years. As such it should be viewed as a social experiment in progress with great positive potential and many inherent dangers. The positive potential of the system is reflected in our ability to answer no to the first study question about perpetuating the negative characteristics of chronic hospital care. Its danger lies in the possibility that pressures of social exclusion and vested-interest politics may force a premature end to the system's development.

Three potential dangers inherent in forcing a premature end to the system's development are (1) the pressure to legitimate system participants or particular types of facilities before we understand their effects in terms of quality of care; (2) our current inability to monitor quality of care in a system of geographically dispersed facilities; and (3) the possibility that closure will result in a return to the state hospital back ward system.

The first danger in forcing a premature end to the development of the sheltered-care system is best illustrated by the volatile political situation in Los Angeles discussed above. Facility operators continually press for the legitimization of their facilities through licensing and zoning decisions. They advocate the establishment of a rotating system as opposed to a selective referral system. Supporting these efforts would ensure the existence of such facilities with limited attention to their role in meeting resident need.

In looking at the second danger, one sees that the absence of an active resident consumer effort makes it extremely difficult to monitor the quality of care in such a large number of facilities. Serious abuse of the former patient does exist in the sheltered-care system, yet, in many respects, the environment is better than what preceded it. This at least is true in terms of resident social functioning. Licensing does not solve the monitoring problem. We need a period of experimentation with several different methods in order to find an adequate solution to the problem of ensuring quality of care.

Finally, those promoting social exclusion by the communities would have the hospital back wards reopened so as to recreate the illusion that mental patients have been entrusted to a benign, protected environment under the best medical care. The assumption that simply sending people back to the community would make them better has proved somewhat erroneous; letting the pendulum swing back the other way will only serve to mask the problem again, not to solve it.

Three potential positive aspects of the system as an aftercare resource involve (1) its visibility, (2) its diversity, (3) its openness to experimentation in the development of new or at least more adequate service models.

The first encouraging aspect of the system in California, as in other parts of the country, is that the community has come face-to-face with its chronically mentally ill. While this has often been the result of muckraking efforts related to the abuse of the former patient in community care, it is extremely important in keeping the needs of this group before the general public.

In the diversity of the multiple approaches to community care employed in these facilities—its second positive aspect—we may find the flexibility to accommodate the great variance in the needs of this population.

Finally, another strength of the system is that, in its current state of flux, it is open to experimentation and the development of new models of aftercare. Small-scale experiments within the current aftercare context can determine, for example, the most effective type of referral system, preferably one which would discourage the continuation of poor-quality facilities while matching the resident to the facility which will best meet his needs. Unfortunately, we must live temporarily with abuses in order to allow room for the development of a truly new and better system of care. This does not mean that such abuse should be ignored. However, the establishment of ex-mental patients in the community and their continued visibility are the best insurance that action will be taken with regard to abuses and that a new and better system of aftercare will be developed.

In any service system too much control can lead to stifling of creativity. The dynamics of sheltered care and its social and political context has promoted the development of a system open to abuse as well as creative activity. Having had an unsatisfactory but stable aftercare situation in the past, we should welcome the possibility of future change.

## References

1. Joint Commission on Mental Illness and Health. *Action for mental health.* New York: Basic Books, 1961.
2. California State Department of Public Welfare. *Handbook on public assistance.*
3. California State Department of Mental Hygiene. *A study of successful treatment.* Sacramento, California: Human Relations Agency, 1972.
4. Hoch Brings Services to Hotel Residents. *Mental Hygiene News.* Albany, New York, State Department of Mental Hygiene, February 28, 1975, p. 6.
5. Morrissey, J. *The case for family care of the mentally ill.* New York: Behavioral Publications, 1967, p. 10.
6. Glasscote, R., Gudeman, J., & Elpers, R. *Halfway houses for the mentally ill.* Washington, D.C.: The Joint Information Service, 1971, p. 15.
7. Segal, S., and Aviram, U. *Factors that facilitate and factors that hinder the reintegration of the mentally ill in their local communities.* Unpublished report to the California State Department of Health, Berkeley, California, 1975, Chap. 5, p. 1.

8. Kramer, M. Statistics of mental disorders in the United States: Current status, some urgent needs and suggested solutions. *Journal of The Royal Statistical Society,* 1969, **132,** 353–407.

9. Barton, R. *Institutional neurosis.* Bristol: Wright, 1959. Wing, J. Institutionalism in mental hospitals. *British Journal of Social and Clinical Psychology,* 1962, **1,** 38–51.

10. Gruenberg, E. Can the reorganization of psychiatric services prevent some cases of social breakdown. In A. Stokes (Ed.), *Psychiatry in transition.* Toronto, Canada: University of Toronto Press, 1966, pp. 95–109.

11. Ellenberger, H. Zoological garden and mental hospital. *Canadian Psychiatric Association Journal,* 1960, 136–47.

12. Wing, J. Institutionalism in mental hospitals. *British Journal of Social and Clinical Psychology,* 1962, **1,** 38–51.

13. Goffman, E. *Asylums.* Bristol, England: Aldine, 1962. Zussman, J. Some explanations of the changing appearance of psychotic patients. In E. Gruenberg (Ed.), *Evaluating the effectiveness of community mental health services.* New York: Milbank Memorial Fund, 1966, pp. 363–94.

14. Cumming, E., & Cumming, J. *Closed ranks.* Cambridge, Massachusetts: Harvard University Press, 1957. Gurin, G., Veroff, J. & Feld, S. *Americans view their mental health: A nationwide interview survey.* Joint Commission on Mental Illness and Health Monograph Series, no. 4. New York: Basic Books, 1960. Nunnally, J. D. *Popular conceptions of mental health: Their development and change.* New York: Holt, 1961.

15. Aviram, U., & Segal, S. Exclusion of the mentally ill: A reflection on an old problem in a new context. *Archives of General Psychiatry,* July 1973, **29,** 126–131.

16. Miller, D. *Worlds that fail, Part I.* Sacramento, California: State Department of Mental Hygiene, 1965.

17. Sososky, L. Putting state mental hospitals out of business—the community approach to treating mental illness in San Mateo County. Berkeley: Graduate School of Public Policy, Memo, 1974.

18. Gulevich, G., & Bourne, P. Mental illness and violence. In D. Daniels, G. Mapshall, & F. Ochberg (Eds.), *Violence and the struggle for existence.* Boston: Little, Brown and Company, 1970, pp. 309–326.

19. *Special study on community care in Santa Clara County.* Sacramento, California: California State Department of Health, 1973.

# III

## Issues in Community Care and the Closing of Hospitals

# 10

# Some Major Issues in the Closing of the Hospitals

MILTON GREENBLATT AND ELIZABETH GLAZIER

Almost all state hospitals in America have undergone a sharp phase-down of inpatient population. A few hospitals have been phased out of existence altogether and some have undergone metamorphosis to facilities serving the retarded or the psychiatric offender, or have been converted to junior colleges or to other such public purposes. As the patients have moved out of the hospitals into the communities, a concomitant improvement in the care and treatment of patients remaining within the hospitals has also ensued. In many institutions this has been quite as remarkable as the community shift itself. These historic, almost revolutionary, changes have brought with them a host of problems of which only a few selected ones can be dealt with in this chapter. These include: the dying hospital, transfer trauma, ghettoization of former mental patients, strategies in the development of satellites, and the narrowing sphere of professional autonomy.

None of these issues has yet been researched in any depth. Since the literature is meager, the authors have had to depend heavily on experience in Massachusetts, particularly the phaseout of Grafton State Hospital, which occurred during the senior author's tenure as commissioner in that state.

MILTON GREENBLATT • Veterans Administration Hospital, Sepulveda, California 91343.     ELIZABETH GLAZIER • Department of Psychiatry, Veterans Administration Hospital, Sepulveda, California 91343.

## The Dying Hospital

Closing of a mental hospital that has been serving the mentally ill of a community for many years is the equivalent of institutional death. In the business world, failures and bankruptcies are familiar, but death of mental hospitals is a relatively new phenomenon in America. In Massachusetts, for example, mental hospitals under state jurisdiction were first established in 1833, the first being Worcester State Hospital in Worcester, Massachusetts, whose birth was pioneered by the eminent Horace Mann, then a member of the Massachusetts legislature. The numbers of hospitals, hospital buildings, and hospitalized patients then increased rapidly until the early 1950s, when the first reversal of trend of inpatient population occurred. However, it was not until 1973 that the first complete phaseout of a hospital in the state of Massachusetts was planned and executed; this was 140 years after the founding of the first state institution.

Expectations and foreboding with respect to possible closing of institutions in America have been building up for years. The downturn of inpatient population that started in the 1950s, and more particularly the *continued* fall in census year by year despite predictions to the contrary by many professionals who thought that the "hard core" of mental patients would halt the trend, were certainly critical factors. The public applause that attended the closing of individual back wards and buildings within giant hospital complexes, and the success in "prevention of hospitalization"[1] for many mental patients in the community, together with the rise of the community mental health movements—all signaled the day when the public would face the actual demise of mental institutions they had long considered a disgrace.

In facing the death of mental hospitals, the community has to deal with complex feelings of loss, relief, and anxiety. Many lives are affected by the closing in many ways. Unfortunately for history, none of these major institutional deaths has been studied and reported with the same detail and sensitivity with which Stotland and Kobler reported.[2] The full meaning of hospital closures will not be appreciated until the human stresses of an institution headed for oblivion are counted against the therapeutic, social, and economic advantages of laying these institutional monuments to rest.

From experience thus far gathered, we can postulate several phases in the sequence of events: (a) mounting anxiety and denial during the phase preceding actual closing operations, with efforts by staff and others to resist, obstruct, and negate planning; (b) rage and depression during the phase when the reality of closing finally dawns on the persons affected; (c) working through of psychological, social, and occupational accommodations necessitated by the closing of the institution; and, finally, (d) adaptation to the new equilibrium with varying degrees of satisfaction or dissatisfaction.

Until detailed dynamics of institutional closures are available, the phases postulated above must be regarded as partly hypothetical.

During the first phase of mounting anxiety and denial, employees, families, and patients contact doctors, superintendents, department heads, legislators, newspapers, etc., asking for information, fearful that the change will visit hardships upon them, and often predicting disaster. Labor groups organize employee resistance to the phaseout, legislators mobilize their political "clout," and patients demonstrate unexpected aggravation of psychotic symptoms, or perhaps develop somatic disease.

During this phase the stresses can be mitigated to some extent by involving, as much as possible, all the affected parties in planning, discussion, sharing of information, and expression of feelings of stress, frustration, depression, anxiety, and loss.

During the second phase, when the reality dawns that final decisions have been made by higher authority despite all that they can do, a feeling of hopelessness overtakes the individuals involved; those who have fought changes bitterly realize that they must bow to public policy. Rage and depression accompany the realization that future options are limited. There is deep concern that the quality of life of family, children, and associates may be impaired. Maintenance of income level, seniority rights in their work relationships, ties with friends and relatives, reimbursement for moving and travel expenses are the major complaints during this period. Again, appropriate representation in decision-making bodies, feedback of essential information to individuals involved, open discussion, assurances regarding salaries, labor rights, etc., and special consideration for hardship cases— these are the major courtesies that management can show staff and families in distress.

The working through of accommodations and adaptations to the new equilibrium are variously handled. Some patients find a better life in the new environment. Ninety percent of Grafton patients, followed up in community placements—i.e., nursing homes, rest homes, or cooperative apartments—preferred those new locations. However, less than 50% of those transferred to other hospitals rated them better than Grafton.[3] Since these were more active treatment hospitals, it is entirely possible that the more active environment was experienced by patients as too stressful for comfort.

Kram[4] recently reported the effects on patient and staff of the closing of a 300-bed clinical and research federal hospital in Lexington, Kentucky, operated since 1935 for the treatment of drug addiction. In February of 1974 the Bureau of Prisons took over that hospital for the rehabilitation of criminal offenders. Kram reports that the patients became apathetic, more resistant to treatment, or acted out. A few of the patients found jobs. For new admissions during the period of phase-down, rehabilitation was compromised by the atmosphere of a dying institution.

The staff reacted with denial, anxiety, disagreements, and reluctance to discharge patients. Depression, feelings of irreversible loss and failure, hopelessness, and lack of confidence bore down upon them. In effect, the death of the hospital was experienced in part as the death of something within them.

## Transfer Trauma

Since major shifts in life adaptation are stressful, we must be concerned with a series of questions related to the trauma of transfer of patients and staff who are dislocated. Are death rates, particularly in the elderly, increased? Are psychosomatic and medical disease aggravated? If so, what are the factors contributing to this increase, and can they be minimized or negated? Preliminary information suggests there may be ways of softening the trauma of transfer and reducing the incidence of death and disability.

Bouriston[5] states that lower death rates occur when patients are well prepared for the move, and are given a choice in the selection and design of facilities to which they will be transferred. Higher death rates are reported where patients have reacted with regression, depression, or denial. Radical changes in life-style were more serious than mild or moderate changes in life-style.

Efforts to reduce the traumatic consequences of relocation should include:

1. Careful attention to physical health, especially of the elderly, with concern for chronic brain syndrome, arteriosclerosis, hypertension, renal disease, arthritis, impairments of memory and sensory apparatus, and liability to systemic infection. Patients with physical disorder are more likely to adapt poorly or not at all to the transfer. All physical deviations, therefore, should be diagnosed and corrected as far as possible.

2. Careful attention to the patient's propensity for confusion, disorientation, anxiety, panic, depression, agitation, and/or increase of delusions and hallucinations in the face of new accommodations forced upon them. These symptoms indicate increased risk of transfer.
3. Psychological and social preparation of both patient and staff for the transfer are important.

The phaseout of Grafton State Hospital in Massachusetts was accomplished by placing Central Office personnel in charge of the overall operation, instead of delegating the closing to local hands. Local management was finding it difficult to make hard decisions that might prove distressing to individuals they had employed for many years. Often they were friends, or even neighbors, of the director. Therefore, all major planning and decisions regarding day-to-day activities were delegated to Central Office psychiatric staff.

During the action part of the phaseout, Drs. Kahn and Kaplan[3] from the Department of Mental Health held daily meetings over a nine-month period with the staff at Grafton. Thereafter they met twice or three times weekly. All findings were reported back to the Department of Mental Health through the deputy commissioner. Thus, a strong link was forged between Central Office and the activities and daily work carried on at the local level. In addition, there were open meetings monthly for discussion and exchange of information for all hospital personnel, as well as a Grafton newsletter that gave weekly information concerning the process of closing. This newsletter explained all decisions or changes in administrative policy and announced which patients would be transferred on any given date.

Patients and kin both were canvassed for their wishes as to which of a number of options they would like to elect. They were asked to indicate their preference for hospital or community—which hospital and what type of facility in the community. The hospital newspaper, in announcing who was leaving each week, gave the staff and patients an opportunity to throw parties where volunteers, nursing personnel, and family members, as well as nurses and other staff from the wards of the new hospital, could attend and say both farewells and welcomes at the same time. The patients got new clothes and personal kits, plus at least $20 from the patient's trust fund, or at least $30 if they were over 65 and were receiving funds from Medicaid. Nurses from Grafton, who knew the patients, accompanied them on their first day of transfer. They informed the new hospital staff of the patients' behavior, and at a later date returned to visit them. It should be noted that personnel had previously taken bus tours to visit the new hospital, and that oftentimes this was the first visit they had ever made to those institutions. With such preparation they could better answer the patient's questions about that hospital, as well as make relationships with the new staff that was to look after their patients.

Personnel also received lectures on the stresses of moving and the importance of preparation to alleviate tension and strain.

Patients were moved in groups of six to ten, together with staff that knew them. The staff that elected to go with patients volunteered for this function. In several hospitals a "Grafton Ward" was established where both the patients and their former staff could continue to be together as a group.

The above is quoted from personal experience to suggest the many forms of humane management of patients that the hospital citizenry felt could be instituted under the prevailing conditions. During the many months of discussion, staff and patients together became deeply involved in innovating ways to soften the blow of separation. In this sense, therefore, Grafton patients received far more attention during the period of their preparation for transfer than they had for years previously.

## Ghettoization

Several authors have indicated that community facilities to receive discharged patients have not been in balance with the requirements of the patients discharged. Although board-and-care homes have increased greatly in California and other states,[6] adequate standards for inspection have not been formulated. These homes, therefore, vary greatly in quality, and many are probably giving the patient less in the way of supervision, support, and freedom than he received in the hospital. The community care of discharged patients has created a new business for small entrepreneurs—attendants, aides, nurses, motel owners—interested in financial return.

Houston and Nelson[7] ask who is responsible for establishing and enforcing standards, and will there be a new Dorothea Dix situation created in the community by the development of many new facilities giving inadequate care.

Boarding homes may turn out to be flophouses. Some patients have been assaulted or victimized by robbers, rapists, or killers. Residual mental illness of many patients makes them less able to defend themselves. Some patients, being chronic sitters, strollers, or shriekers, invite attack. Patients may roam the streets, or remain isolated in their rooms. Welfare payments, on which they depend, may be low. Stewart and colleagues[8] call for clearly defined standards for all foster homes, and training programs for foster home directors. Wolpert and Wolpert[9] state that under current conditions there is a definitely increased risk of physical illness and mortality.

The lack of facilities is further compounded by lack of rigorous bases for determining what facilities are most beneficial or where the facility should be sited. The great opportunity, therefore, for research in comparative effectiveness of aftercare modalities for selected patient groups is still to be grasped.

The community's reaction to the vastly increased numbers of mentally ill within its ranks is still developing. Some major trends are beginning to emerge. There is increased community sensitivity to "bizarre" and "threatening" behavior, and increased demands for rehospitalization. At the same time, advocacy on behalf of released patients is growing and in some quarters tolerance and acceptance has increased. In setting up halfway houses or community homes in Massachusetts, hard opposition came mainly from plush suburban areas. Communities that reacted with opposition expressed fears that the patients would create "scenes," such as urinating in public, running naked through the streets, frightening children, or bringing drugs into the neighborhood. Zoning regulations and fire safety codes were invoked to prevent the setting up or use of facilities for postdischarged patients. The Belle-Terre Decision of the Supreme Court and the Long Beach municipal rulings are two such legal maneuvers used to prevent patients' entry into "good" communities. Fear of reduction in value of property is often behind the hard resistance manifested.

Segal,[6] who studied 214 facility operators and 400 residents (reported in this volume), indicated that 19% of facility operators received complaints from neighbors, 14% received complaints which were conveyed to local authorities, and 4% were threatened or harassed by neighbors. Forty percent of facility operators said that at least one of their residents had been picked up by the police in the last year, only one of which was for a violent act. Only 4% of police contacts involved bizarre behavior. The most frequent reason for being picked up was for being "lost" and wandering around the neighborhood.

The fact that a number of persons with a history of mental treatment, however, have committed violent crimes with subsequent outcry from the public, the press, and legislative investigators has substantially slowed the process of reentry of former patients into the community and, in the long run, has encouraged ghettoization.[9]

Many other factors have, in fact, contributed to the ghettoization of the mentally ill. Often the family has closed ranks against the mentally ill person and actively opposed his return to the community; or the patient, in fact, has no family to go to. Restrictive zoning ordinances or safety codes, as already mentioned, are a serious impediment. Dependence of the patient on welfare at the subsistence level often means gravitation to subsistence communities; and the presence of boarding and rooming homes in low socioeconomic neighborhoods encourages the accumulation of patients in those areas. Finally, lack of standards for licensing or inspection of facilities further accelerates the process of ghettoization.

A prime example of ghettoization and its consequences is described in San Jose, California, by Wolpert and Wolpert. Some 1,100 patients released from hospitals during a fifteen-year period concentrated in this college town, which possessed 74% of the available unlicensed board-and-care facilities of the county. Operators of board-and-care homes were untrained. Follow-up of patients was inadequate. Jobs for patients were lacking. Patients funds were scarce.

Happily, a silver lining appeared to brighten this sorry situation: A community of students organized under strong leadership to provide human and material assistance to some 700 of the residents in 22 homes.

The lesson of San Jose must be taken seriously as a commentary on the excesses of the community mental health movement. In general there is relatively little objection to the basic philosophy of comprehensive community mental health care, and in practice thousands of patients unsuitable for continuing hospitalization have been released, while thousands of others have been prevented from unnecessary hospitalization. However—although most would agree that the treatment of the patient earlier in his clinical course, closer to his home, without disruption of ties to family, community, or job, is a principle of undeniable importance—in some states this fine principle has been virtually invalidated by unfortunate dumping of patients into communities ill prepared to receive them.

One interesting positive plan to deal with the problems of community adaptation is reported by Oberleder.[10] Bronx Hospital in New York closed its doors to the elderly whose difficulties were either physical, social, or economic, and for whom state hospitalization would function more as a cause, than as a cure, of mental illness. However, Bronx Hospital took the responsibility for doing something in the community through the medium of mobile geriatric teams, family consultation, and day hospital. It offered education and supervision in the management of geriatric patients on the spot in the community, including seminars, reality therapy, visits to other hospitals by staff, and mobilization of visiting nurse services.

Some 35 facilities availed themselves of the hospital consultation program for the elderly. Oberleder found that fear, anger, and frustration were the bases of almost all bizarre behavioral episodes. There was a high correlation between a diagnosis of acute or chronic brain syndrome and socioeconomic or relocation stresses. It was the poor, the lonely, and the uneducated, in the end, who generally succumbed.

## Strategies in Development of Satellite Facilities

A critical factor in developing a proper balance between the phasedown and phaseout of inpatient facilities, and phaseup of community alternatives, has to do with the technology of the development of such facilities.

In a country as diverse as ours, there is marked variation in strategy depending upon what agency initiates the action, the client population served, the financial mechanism used, the public reaction to the siting of health facilities in their areas, and the response of immediate neighbors to the facility. While a great deal of experience has accumulated in the last few decades, there are few systematic studies to guide us at this point.

The stimulus for the development of a community facility may come from the community, from the local mental hospital, from the county or state Department of Mental Health, or a combination of these.

In Massachusetts a community was regarded as "ready" for a mental health facility when it became aware of its needs; mobilized important elements in the community, such as legislators, mayors, mental health and retardation leaders; selected a site; raised funds for a secretary; and purchased or rented property for which maintenance was provided. All this was done on a voluntary basis, although often departmental officials played a role in contacting citizen leaders explaining need and defining community roles. When local interest and cooperation was high and no major stumbling blocks were in the way, the local group asked for departmental funds for staff, and, when this was granted, entered into an agreement with the commissioner of mental health defining the "partnership." This method had the advantage that interest stemmed essentially from the citizens themselves and the department avoided hassles and stresses arising out of local opposition or resistance.

The disadvantages were that it sometimes required years for local citizens to band together and to assemble the resources necessary. Applications for state personnel were not regularly matched by formula, but depended upon legislative response to annual departmental recommendations. Also, communities that were "ready" were not necessarily those of greatest need, although departmental consultants did try to stimulate communities of highest priority.

In other states, as in California, an important incentive is the predictability of state matching, which may be as high as 90%, to a 10% raise by local groups. In addition, specific financial reward results from providing local treatment of mentally ill patients in the community rather than referring them to state hospitals. Thus, California's state and county hospital population has been reduced to 75 beds per 100,000 population,[11] which is regarded as on the low side for developed states; as a consequence, four major hospitals have been closed.

In many instances hospitals themselves provide both the rationale and the wherewithal for community satellites through decentralization or unitization of their services and the assignment of each service to a defined geographic area. The philosophy of outreach and the responsibility for a catchment area is thus stimulated. Staff soon finds ways to develop outpatient satellites, both as a means of preventing unnecessary admissions and as a means of follow-up of discharged patients and prevention of readmission.

In the VA system, using Sepulveda in the San Fernando Valley as an example,[12] the decentralization of psychiatric services into five components, each serving the veterans of a defined geographic area of the San Fernando Valley, was recently initiated. This quickly gave rise to six satellites serving discharged veterans as well as nonhospitalized veterans early in their clinical course, closer to their homes, without the necessity to disrupt ties to family, community, or job. Siting of satellites for this VA system turned out to be a comparatively easy job as the built-in constituency of the American Legion Posts throughout the valley generously supplied space, utilities, and volunteers to help this hospital with its outreach.

Concerning the strategies of establishing satellites, Crawford and Wolpert[13] studied 15 controversial site decisions in Pennsylvania between 1969 and 1973. Eight of these were finally implemented. The study was aimed at determining what factors favored or retarded success. Facilities were more likely to be established if they were sited in the inner city on the fringe of commercial activities, or in suburban areas where zoning variances were not obstructive. They were also likely to succeed if situated away from schools or playgrounds. Controversy arose most in relation to lower-middle-class neighborhoods. Success was association with community involvement in planning and in the determination of the functions and services to be offered. It was best if the mental health officials painted a realistic rather than a glowing picture of the benefits, and undertook operations with as little fanfare as possible. Patterns of community organization to be avoided included playing off one part of the community against another, involving the community in controversy before the courts, and placing undue reliance on the persuasive testimony of experts.

## The Narrowing Sphere of Professional Autonomy

As the citizens and the legislature become more interested and involved in the plight of the mentally ill, administrators of hospitals and executives of health care systems are being held more and more accountable for the type of services provided. Recently citizens and the legislators have made powerful inroads on the autonomy of superintendents of hospitals and of schools for the retarded. Accountability to state and federal bodies regulating care practices is now required for Medicare, Medicaid, and maternal and child health reimbursements. Administrators are accountable to accreditation bodies also for a mountain of details related to safety, living arrangements, and programs. To this have been added new standards of care and treatment arising from court actions, and from the legislature, based on revision and recodification of laws related to the rights of the mentally ill.

This shift in balance of control from the professionals to the legislature and the public has been dramatized in some of the phaseouts of mental hospitals. In the case of phasing out of Grafton Hospital we were forced to negotiate with members of the Ways and Means Committee for many months before permission was obtained to close that hospital. This was a hospital which the governor and the commissioner, after much study, felt must be closed as soon as possible because of very poor physical plants, inadequate water supply, semirural situation, difficulty in recruiting qualified staff, and uninspired programs.

For each step toward final closure clearance had to be obtained from officials of Ways and Means.

The commissioner of mental health *did* possess the power at that time to move *patients* from one facility to another. This power in Massachusetts had been exercised with relative freedom for many decades. But the legislature had withheld the power to move *staff* from one facility or institution to another. Total evacuation of a hospital that had been standing for more than 70 years was regarded as a phenomenon of such far-reaching implications that responsible legislators felt they should watch the Department of Mental Health carefully, ready to use their authority to control possible precipitous action of the department.

The commissioner's control of his own department was in the balance. By statute he could move patients, but if this were done without the agreement of powerful legislators, all actions toward closure could be easily stopped by legislative mandate. (This subsequently occurred in the state of California, after several hospitals were phased out.) The great fear of legislators was that employees would be laid off or suffer undue hardships due to change of residence, loss of friends, disruption of children's schooling, or the loss of a second job by a family member.

Finally, by exercising his power to move patients to situations with greater therapeutic potential, the commissioner slowly reduced the inpatient population at Grafton. As a result, per diem costs began to rise to potentially embarrassing levels. The legislators realized that Grafton would soon be left with lots of personnel tending very few patients at astronomical costs.

The point of this example is that the balance of power between mental health agencies and the legislature, always a background issue, is now being fought out on the battleground of the closing of state hospitals. More than one state legislature has indicated its interest in expanding its regulation of both treatment and research in mental health, including ECT, psychosurgery, drug therapy, and behavior modification—and now the closing of hospitals.

In effect the legislature, and sometimes the courts, have undertaken to prescribe the modalities of therapy they endorse and the limits of therapeutic application. Only time will tell where the new professional–legislative equilibrium will settle down and how this will eventually impact upon patient care and treatment.

## References

1. Greenblatt, M., Moore, R. F., Albert, R. S., & Solomon, M. H. *The prevention of hospitalization.* New York: Grune and Stratton, 1963.
2. Stotland, E., & Kobler, A. L. *Life and death of a mental hospital.* Seattle: University of Washington Press, 1965.
3. Kahn, N. A., & Kaplan, R. M. Personal communication from follow-up of Grafton patients.

4. Kram, L. Closing an institution: Its effect on patients and on staff. *Hospital and Community Psychiatry*, April 1975, **26** (4).
5. Bouriston, N., Pastalan, L. A., Tars, S. *Some important concepts on the study of forced relocation.* Presented at annual meeting of Gerontological Society, Houston, Texas, Oct. 29, 1971.
6. Segal, S. Life in board and care: Its political and social context. Proceeding of a Conference on the Closing of State Mental Hospitals, Plog Research, Inc. and Stanford Research Inst., April, 1974.
7. Houston, P. E., Nelson, R. L. Are state hospitals passé? *Medical World News Review*, October 1974, **1**(2).
8. Stewart, H., Lafave, H. G., Grunberg, F., & Herjanic, M. Problems in phasing out a large public psychiatric hospital. *American Journal of Psychiatry*, July 1968, **125**(I).
9. Wolpert, J., & Wolpert, E. The relocation of released mental hospital patients into residential communities. SRI Report, April, 1974. (Mimeo)
10. Oberleder, M. A state hospital closes its doors to the elderly. *Gerontology*, Spring, 1973.
11. Statistical Note 98, Biometry Branch, NIMH, November, 1973.
12. Personal experience of the senior author.
13. Crawford, R., & Wolpert, J. *The siting of mental health satellite facilities: Demonstration of a comparative case study instrument.* Unpublished paper, June, 1974.

# 11

# Moving Patients Out of Hospitals—In Whose Interest?

JONAS ROBITSCHER

No one would argue that state mental hospitals in the United States have fulfilled any kind of promise of providing a therapeutic atmosphere for the mentally ill. Or is it their purpose to provide a therapeutic atmosphere? Does furnishing a custodial milieu provide sufficient benefits for some patients who would be worse off without the hospital so that their commitment seems justifiable? Until recently no one could be found to say a good word for the state mental hospital system; now that we are beginning to see the results of new policies that restrict the use of state hospitals, many people are beginning to see the state hospital system as preferable to moving disturbed and incompetent people out into the community.

Before we can decide how badly state hospitals function and plan what they must do to change, we must decide what the purpose is of the state mental hospital. A literature has developed which states that these hospitals are society's way of segregating those who make society uncomfortable, that the mental health system has not been concerned with the best interests of the patient but instead has been society's

JONAS ROBITSCHER • Emory University School of Law, Atlanta, Georgia 30322.

agent.[1] Some commentators writing in this tradition see no reason for involuntary commitment.*

Another line of literature tells us that hospitals do have a purpose but they have not been fulfilling that purpose, that inadequate concern for patients has deprived them of their opportunity to regain their mental health to the degree which would entitle them to be released. The concept of the right to treatment is that the liberty which patients are deprived of in the course of an involuntary commitment must be paid for by the state in terms of a high grade of psychiatric care.[2]

In recent years stimulated by the concept that patients should be treated in the community, an addition to this concept has developed, that state hospitalization should be used only exceedingly sparingly when it has been demonstrated that the patient cannot function even when supported by a wide range of community services. Those who hold this view, a popular view at this time, are willing to siphon off money and personnel from the state hospital system to use for community mental health, so the right to treatment, although supported in principle, is not always seen as a rationale for attempting to improve the quality of state hospital care.[3]

Still another point of view represented in the literature, the more traditional approach to the question, is that patients who are involuntarily committed to state hospitals are receiving a benefit by the very fact of their commitment—the custodial care they receive may be far from optimal care but still may represent something better than a denial of care which would result if free and low-cost hospitalization were not available. The care that is given is funded by the legislature and it is in the power of the legislature to provide services at a lower level than that which would be provided by private mental hospitals. Custodial care is seen as a legitimate function of state hospitals.

The argument can be made that as bad as most state hospitals are and as much as they should be upgraded, they have still served a function in providing a safe place for incompetents who would otherwise not fare well in complex modern society. But the reformers who wish to produce an overnight change in the state hospital system either by upgrading it beyond all recognition (a consummation devoutly to be wished but one that some commentators think can come only from an evolutionary process that stems from the institutions, not from reform imposed by outside forces) or by blasting the system out of existence

---

*When the American Association for the Abolition of Involuntary Hospitalization was formed in 1970, its directors included Thomas Szasz and Erving Goffman, sociologist and author of *Asylums* (New York: Doubleday, 1961).

(by abolishing involuntary commitments and by making hospitalization a rare phenomenon) are not ready to see apologists for the system as men of goodwill. The reformers see traditional hospital personnel as the enemy and legal activism as the means to carry the war to them.

Three important movements in mental health have come together to create a situation in which legal activism can force large numbers of patients out of the state hospital system: (1) the rise of the community mental health movement, (2) legal restrictions on admission to and length of stay in mental hospitals, and (3) legal acceptance of a constitutional right to treatment. The most recent and most visible is the concept of the right to treatment, which has caused many hospitals to push patients out of the state hospital system so that a better quality of care, one that might come up to a constitutionally guaranteed minimum standard of treatment, can be provided for those patients who are retained. But before the right to treatment surfaced, the community mental health center concept, which argued that outpatient care in the community should be stressed rather than state hospital care, and legal attacks of commitment practices, which have forced hospitals to be more selective in admissions and readier to let patients go, paved the way for the attack on the state hospital system.

Morton Birnbaum, the general practitioner–lawyer who single-handedly and single-mindedly developed the idea that hidden in the Constitution was a new right that could be enforced to improve the lot of state mental patients, has always emphasized two points which are now in danger of being ignored. The first is that the task of defining what is acceptable psychiatric treatment is so technical and so ill-suited to the judicial decision-making process that courts should steer clear of this task; instead, they should only promulgate a few simple guidelines (one of the first that he suggested was equality of staff–patient ratios in state mental hospitals with ratios in accredited private hospitals) and they should never go into the more complicated specifics of treatment plans and programs. The second Birnbaum precept was that in spite of the potential usefulness of a court-recognized and court-implemented constitutionally guaranteed right to treatment, the state legislature, which is the only branch of government that "has the means to set up a comprehensive scheme and to coordinate it with necessary legislative appropriations" rather than the judiciary, "seems the proper instrumentality to establish a realistic right to treatment."[4]

Birnbaum did feel that without a Supreme Court mandate, legislatures would not act: "Unfortunately, however, until recently it seemed a fact of life that neither the Congress nor any state legislature would take it upon itself to deal with this problem unless the Supreme Court recognized a realistic right to treatment." But he saw the legislative approach as the real answer to the plight of the state mental hospital patient.

*Wyatt* v. *Stickney,*\* a 1971 Federal District Court case in Alabama, held that there is such a right; in November 1974, the United States Circuit Court of Appeals for the Fifth Circuit unanimously affirmed the ruling.† Eventually the Supreme Court will have to decide if there is indeed a constitutional right to treatment for the civilly committed mental patient which allows the court to set hospital standards and to maintain supervision over hospitals in order to enforce these standards, or possibly if courts should intervene in the mental health system on the basis of some other rationale, for example, to see that alternative facilities are provided so that the holding can be as little restricted as possible. But the Supreme Court has not been anxious to enter this field of controversy.

Birnbaum's injunctions to limit judicial intervention into state hospital administration and to rely on the legislative route rather than the judicial route to secure improved hospitals have not been heeded by the *Wyatt* courts, and as a result we are in trouble. Birnbaum himself recognizes that his method of securing help for state mental hospital patients is capable of jumping the tracks. He said at a 1974 meeting:

> At present . . . it is really impossible to do more than speculate as to whether its present paths are definitely leading to better or worse psychiatric and other medical care in our state mental hospitals. I can only say now what I have repeatedly stressed before, that this concept has a potential both for use and abuse; perhaps this is a characteristic of almost all needed social reforms. In the future it can lead almost *anywhere* and do almost anything as far as altering the needed care given to state mental hospital patients.
>
> Realistically, of course, it may do nothing for the patient while taking up quite a bit of the time of our courts and increasing state mental hospital expenditures. Or hopefully, it may be the dawn of a new day for the state mental hospital as a vital, integral and necessary part of the therapeutic mental health continuum. Or it may cause the state mental hospital to be, even more than today, the wastebasket for the chronic severely mentally ill from the community and from the community mental health facilities unwilling or unable to manage these individuals.[5]

Birnbaum could have added another possibility. The concept may lead to a sudden great constriction of the state hospital system so that fewer patients will be treated in these hospitals and those patients who are treated will be released much sooner, and this has the potentiality for both good and bad.

\**Wyatt* v. *Stickney,* 325 F. Supp. 781 (M.D. Ala. 1971); 334 F. Supp. 1341 (M.D. Ala. 1971); 344 F. Supp. 373, 387 (M.D. Ala. 1972).
†*Wyatt* v. *Aderholt,* 503 F.2d 1305 (5th Cir. 1974).

Still another possibility is that it will force the expenditure of so much money to bring state hospitals up to court-ordered standards that mental health dollars will not be available for many other purposes, including the care in the community that is the goal of those who are most opposed to state hospital care; in that case the mental health system will not be allowed to develop through a process of growth and change dictated by the needs of patients but will have to conform to the pattern imposed by courts. And that brings us back to the question of whether court proceedings are the best mechanism for the hammering out of mental health policy.

The move to enforce a right to treatment for state mental hospital patients is not always pushed as a means of helping state hospital patients; the concept can be used for other ends. *Wyatt* v. *Stickney* was originally brought not in the interests of patients but in the interests of personnel.

As the appeals court which affirmed the decision in *Wyatt* v. *Aderholt* said: "This case began innocuously enough, when a cut in the Alabama cigarette tax forced the state to fire 99 professional, subprofessional, and intern employees at the Bryce Hospital, a state-run institution for the mentally ill at Tuscaloosa."* The case was brought in behalf of three patients, representative of the class of patients, and five of the recently terminated employees, representative of the class of 99 employees who had been dismissed for budgetary reasons.

The complaint did not allege that conditions had been bad at Bryce or that patients' rights had been violated before the termination of these employees. It alleged merely that the employees had been discharged entirely for budgetary reasons, that the rights of the employees to hold their jobs were being violated since they had not had notice and a hearing, and that as a result of the discharge the patients at Bryce would not receive adequate treatment.

In a later phase of *Wyatt* v. *Stickney* the case became more truly oriented to the rights of the patients, not the personnel—although the rights of these two classes often run together. In later stages of the case the employee plaintiffs disappeared from the case and representatives of the class of patients at the other Alabama hospital for the mentally ill and of the state facility for the mentally retarded were added. The court then found that many of the basic conditions which prevailed at these three facilities indicated that they were being operated in a constitutionally impermissible manner.

As the case progressed some—but not all—of the lawyers for the

*Wyatt* v. *Aderholt.*

hospital patients stated that their main interest was not to improve these three facilities. The purpose of the suit according to these lawyers—who were possibly not representative of the thinking that guided the case but whose views are still significant—was to "bomb" the state mental hospital system out of existence. Judge Johnson had found that there was a constitutionally guaranteed right to treatment, that patients "involuntarily committed through noncriminal procedures and without the constitutional protections that are afforded defendants in criminal proceedings" are "committed for treatment purposes" and as a result they "unquestionably have a constitutional right to receive such individual treatment as will give each of them a realistic opportunity to be cured or to improve his or her mental condition."* It followed that great changes would have to be made in every phase of the hospitals' running—its physical plant, its ratio of staff to patients, its standard of personnel, its ability to provide less restrictive alternatives than involuntary hospitalization, its policies on use of patient labor, and many more. Let us press this case and force these changes, so said some lawyers, not because we really want to secure better hospitals and better treatment in these hospitals but to make the cost of care per day per patient so expensive that mental hospitals will be forced to close their doors. Then patients will be treated in the community, in community mental health centers, which, said these lawyers, is where they will receive the best and most humane treatment. The result of the case could then be not the improvement of the lot of the involuntarily state hospital committed patient but the abolition of involuntary commitments, the extinction of the class of patient the case was ostensibly brought to help.

Another possibility is a classic confrontation between the judiciary asserting it has the power to impose change and the legislative and administrative branches of government. The enforcement measures that the court in the *Wyatt* case asserts are possibilities that could lead to a redistribution of the powers of government, a departure from a present balance of power achieved through a system of checks and balances that works partly by the limitation of the judiciary of its own power to interfere and control. The very real possibility exists, then, that the right-to-treatment concept may not only not benefit the state mental hospital patient to the extent that Birnbaum originally hoped, but that it may actually harm some patients and at the same time the concept may damage the constitutional system.

A series of complicated legal developments has robbed the right-

---

*Wyatt v. *Stickney,* 325 F. Supp. 781 (M.D. Ala. 1971).

to-treatment concept of some of its legal authority, but strangely enough that has not stopped the spread of the concept and its increased acceptance by institutional psychiatrists.

An understanding of the present status of the right to treatment involves references to the Supreme Court's position (or more appropriately, refusal to take a position) on the issue, to the many similar cases that are now being brought in other jurisdictions, and to alternative legal theories which are being called into use to bolster up the theory of Birnbaum that involuntary detention places a requirement on the state to furnish treatment of a quality that can be judicially determined and judicially enforced.

Before the Fifth Circuit Court of Appeals decided the *Wyatt* case, it had foreshadowed its endorsement of the concept of the right to treatment in the case of *Donaldson* v. *O'Connor*.* In that case, a patient for almost fifteen years at Florida's Chattahoochee State Hospital sued two psychiatrists, claiming that he had not received treatment during his holding and he had had a constitutional right to treatment. The Court of Appeals called this a "novel and important question" and came out with an unequivocal pronouncement: "We hold that a person involuntarily civilly committed to a state mental hospital has a constitutional right to receive such individual treatment as will give him a reasonable opportunity to be cured or to improve his mental condition. † This case was appealed to the United States Supreme Court. The Supreme Court avoided the question of right to treatment in its decision in *O'Connor* v. *Donaldson*‡ and it went out of its way to not only avoid ruling on the issue but to deprive the ruling of the circuit court of its value as a precedent in other right-to-treatment cases. The Supreme Court decided that the case could be decided in favor of the patient's right to liberty by dealing only with the question of whether the harmlessly mentally ill can be held against their wills in simple custodial confinement. Donaldson had a right to be released, the Court said, but it did not rule on whether he had a right to treatment. In deciding that a state may not constitutionally confine in a custodial facility a nondangerous person who is capable of surviving on the outside, the Supreme Court—not surprisingly—embraced a dangerousness criterion as the standard for commitment. But this has nothing to do with the right to treatment. It does not tell us whether nondangerous patients who get meaningful treatment can be retained or whether dangerous patients

---

*Donaldson* v. *O'Connor*, 493 F.2d 507 (5th Cir. 1974).
†Ibid., at 520.
‡*O'Connor* v. *Donaldson*, 422 U.S. 563 (1975).

who get no treatment can be retained. It tells us no more than we knew already—and had known for decades—concerning the rights of mental patients. Some commentators have suggested that the importance of the *Donaldson* decision, if it is important, is that it is the first case in which the Supreme Court has granted plenary review to consider the constitutional rights of civilly committed mental patients.

The Supreme Court appeared to view as a threat to liberty the instruction to the jury issued by the trial judge and approved by the circuit court, that "the purpose of involuntary hospitalization is treatment and not mere custodial care or punishment if a patient is not a danger to himself of others." In his concurring opinion, Chief Justice Burger rejects this quid pro quo justification for the involuntary hospitalization of the nondangerous and he points out that the decision of the Supreme Court offers no support whatsoever for the doctrine of a constitutional right to treatment.* In Justice Stewart's opinion for the court, it is specifically stated that the decision deprives the court of appeals judgment of precedential effect.†

The cases in which the right to treatment are a central concept, *Wyatt* v. *Stickney* and *Burnham* v. *Department of Public Health*,‡ which were decided by the fifth circuit in favor of the right, will never be ruled upon by the Supreme Court. The state of Alabama decided not to appeal the decision against it; it preferred to work out an accommodation with the attorneys representing the patients. The state of Georgia, in the *Burnham* case, asked for the Supreme Court review, but certiorari was denied.§

In the meantime right-to-treatment cases are being brought in a great many jurisdictions, and these deal not only with mental hospitals but with youth correctional facilities, institutions for the retarded, and other holding facilities. Many institutions are using *Wyatt* standards to upgrade their services—sometimes at the expense of part of their patient load, which they discharge in order to provide better care for patients that are left—although they are not in the area of the fifth circuit (Alabama, Florida, Georgia, Louisiana, Mississippi, and Texas).

In the Willowbrook case, *New York State Association for Retarded Children, Inc.* v. *Rockefeller,* ‖ the court used instead of the right-to-treatment rationale a somewhat different concept, that the residents at

*Ibid., at 580 and 585.
†Ibid., at 577–578, n. 12.
‡*Burnham* v. *Department of Public Health*, 503 F.2d 1319 (5th Cir. 1974).
§*Burnham* v. *Department of Public Health*, cert den. 422 U.S. 1057 (1975).
‖ *New York State Association for Retarded Children, Inc.*, v. *Rockefeller*, 357 F. Supp. 752 (E.D. N.Y. 1973).

Willowbrook had a right to freedom from harm, a right that had previously been found for prison inmates held under cruel conditions. In a later development in the same case the court said, referring to *Wyatt:* "Somewhat different legal rubrics have been employed in these cases—'protection from harm' in this case and 'right to treatment' and 'need for care' in others. It appears there is no bright line separating these standards."*

A case with more potential for shaking up the mental health establishment than Wyatt is *Dixon* v. *Weinberger,*† the St. Elizabeth's Hospital case, brought against the hospital, the National Institute of Mental Health which runs the hospital, and the District of Columbia. The ruling depends on the rationale of *Lake* v. *Cameron,*‡ in which Judge David Bazelon set forth a doctrine of "least restrictive alternative," stating that "deprivation of liberty solely because of the dangers to the ill persons themselves should not go beyond what is necessary for their protection."§ (The requirement of a holding in the "least restrictive alternative" had been part of the *Wyatt* case order, but it had not been emphasized because it was overshadowed by the idea of a constitutional treatment right.) Although it applies only to the District of Columbia, the case will be followed by similar suits in other jurisdictions. The court has required that the defendants establish a network of suitable community-based facilities for mental patients now inappropriately confined in St. Elizabeth's. An attorney in the case has estimated that 1,000 of the 2,200 inpatients in the hospital would be eligible for placement in other less restrictive facilities—intermediate and skilled-care nursing homes, foster homes, personal care homes, halfway houses, and room and board facilities.[6] Whether good community resources will be developed or whether more patients will be diagnosed as not committable and left to their own devices will be seen as this and similar cases develop.

The same neglect of patients that motivated the right-to-treatment cases of the 1970s had been the impetus in the 1960s for the extension of the mental health system into the community. The scandal of mental hospitals which provided only the most meager kind of custodial care demanded action, but the action when it came did not solve the problem. The Community Mental Health Centers Act of October, 1963, enlarged the scope of psychiatric activity, redefined many problems

*New York State Association for Retarded Children, Inc., v. Carey,* 393 F. Supp. 715, 719 (E.D. N.Y. 1974).
†*Dixon* v. *Weinberger,* 405 F. Supp. 974 (D.D.C. Dec. 23, 1975).
‡*Lake* v. *Cameron,* 364 F.2d 657 (D.C. Cir. 1966).
§Ibid., at 660.

which had previously been seen as social problems as psychiatric and thus medical problems, and instead of directly addressing the plight of the state hospital patient by insisting on the improvement of hospitals proposed to help the patient in another way, by making it possible for him to avoid the hospital or spend less time in the hospital. It proposed a new philosophy of care: "The objective of modern treatment of persons with major mental illness is to enable the patient to maintain himself in the community in a normal manner." This was the response of Congress to the message that President Kennedy had sent eight months earlier, the first presidential message ever to deal directly with the mental health movement: "We need a new kind of health facility, one which will return mental health care to the mainstream of American medicine and at the same time upgrade mental health service."[7]

Mandatory or "essential" psychiatric services, which had to be provided by community mental health centers to qualify them for federal assistance, were provided in the community. Since the existing facilities for the most part were removed from the community, the new policy meant that the services—inpatient, outpatient, partial hospitalization, emergency, and consultation and educational—would now reach many who had not previously had psychiatric services but that there would be a diversion of money, personnel, and attention from existing hospitals that were not located so that they could fit into the community scheme. The state hospital patient who could be followed in the community would be benefited providing that he could be given enough attention and support so that he could maintain himself well in the community, and some potential state hospital patients might be able to avoid hospitalization. But seriously disturbed and chronic patients might not benefit from this program—and we have heard much criticism indicating that in fact to a large extent they have not benefited. The new policy would also cause other complexities. It emphasized prevention—although many critics of psychiatry do not think psychiatric entities are well enough defined so they can be identified after they happen, let alone before they happen (see Ennis & Litwack[1])—and the process of prevention meant that a wide net would have to be cast that would pick up not only that class of patients who otherwise would migrate to the state hospital but many other patients whose pathology might or might not have led to hospitalization. By extending the scope of treatment to so many new prospective patients, psychiatrists and psychologists would have to act more in a supervisory role and the actual therapy would have to be in charge of paraprofessionals. The relationship of psychiatrists and psychologists to these new treatment providers would have to be defined—and the process of definition and redefinition, only recently well under way, has proven to be complicated and painful. The question of third-party payments for medical care when much of the treatment is not being provided by psychiatrists and psychologists remains to be worked out. Nevertheless, psychiatry in the community mental health movement has set up a new front, and to support this front money and personnel have been diverted from the state mental hospital system.

This diversion of support has accelerated with the advent of the franchised mental hospital, run for profit, and with greater emphasis on psychiatric care in the general hospital; the short-term, good-prognosis patient, the affluent and insurance-covered patient is diverted into these treatment locales and is supported there at a high cost per day. The money spent at these facilities is not available for the shoring up of the state mental hospital system. The state mental hospital system, the "second-class" system, is left to care for the poor, the uninsured, the chronic, and the unmanageable patient, and only a few in these categories are able to pay their own way or to have it paid for them by any other agency beside the state itself.

It would not be reasonable to expect patients to patronize state hospitals by choice in many jurisdictions; although the cost of running a mental hospital does not always correlate directly with the quality of care it offers, it would not be reasonable to expect that the $9.99 a day that Mississippi spends per patient or the $11.18 a day that South Carolina spends or the $14.06 that Virginia spends would provide facilities that would attract affluent patients.[8] Even when patients could be reimbursed by a third party for the cost of their hospitalization, the fact that the state hospitals are not accredited keeps the state from recovering funds.

Morton Birnbaum has stated that by 1965, the year when Medicaid was first enacted, it was demonstrably true that a two-tier system of care and treatment was being provided for the hospitalized mentally ill. The lower tier, which made up the majority of the hospitalized mentally ill, consisted of the sicker and poorer patients. "Those patients were receiving grossly inadequate care and treatment in underfinanced, overcrowded and understaffed state mental hospitals, in buildings that were frequently antiquated and often were health and fire hazards. Funds for these state mental institutions came almost entirely from state governments. The funds provided by the patients and their families were so minimal that realistically speaking they could be considered nonexistent."

He contrasts this with the upper tier, a smaller number of patients including the less sick and the more wealthy. "They usually received adequate care and treatment in well-financed, physically adequate and fully staffed nonpublic mental hospitals. Funds for these facilities came from the patients and their families, from charitable contributions by members of the community and from various federal, state and local governmental sources."[9]

Birnbaum felt that under Medicaid sharing formulas, which provided that 75% of the cost of Medicaid disbursements by the state would be reimbursed by the federal government, it would be possible to upgrade the *Wyatt* case hospitals if the state hospitals were improved to meet federal standards and if there was a successful challenge of the constitutionality of the Medicaid exclusion of state mental patients under 65. George Dean, who had become chief counsel for the *Wyatt* case plaintiffs, at first agreed and then decided against challenging the Medicaid exclusion, according to Birnbaum. His argument was that the state mental institution system was basically bad and should be done away with in favor of alternative community facilities.

Morton Birnbaum decided on a new approach; he brought an action, which was unsuccessful, in New York* to combat the inequity between the two tiers of mental hospital care. Birnbaum argued that when a poor patient goes to a state mental hospital, no federal money goes to improving hospital care, but when a "less sick, wealthier, probably white and voluntarily hospitalized patient" enters a nonstate mental hospital, Medicaid money is used to reimburse the private hospital. The suit asked that the benefits of Medicaid be extended to state mental hospitals, at a potential annual cost of $1.5 billion of additional Medicaid funds, or that alternatively the entire Medicaid statute be declared unconstitutional. Birnbaum found at this time that his former allies in his fight for the right to treatment no longer were with him in this case; he feels that they believed, as did George Dean, that the state mental hospital system should be abolished and that increased funding would only perpetuate an evil.[10]

A three-judge district court ruled unanimously that the Medicaid exclusion was a rational discrimination for Congress to make; the judges did not consider the issue which had been raised that was ruled to be so important in the *Wyatt* case, that the involuntariness of the commitment placed a special burden on the state to provide a reasonable level of care.

The degree of support Birnbaum received from legal activists in one case and not in the other is corroboration, along with other evi-

*Legion v. Richardson, 354 F. Supp. 456 (S.D., N.Y. 1973); aff'd sub nom Legion v. Weinberger, 414 U.S. 1058 (1973); petition for rehearing denied 415 U.S. 939 (1974).

dence such as the statements of *Wyatt* case counsel, that some of the proponents of the right to treatment do not want state mental hospital facilities improved.

Two factors in the reduction of the census rolls of the state mental hospitals have been explored; the emphasis on the right to treatment which raises hospital standards so that more care must be given which often can be accomplished only by offering this more care to fewer patients; and the growth of the community mental health movement which stresses outpatient care. A third important factor is judicial emphasis on stricter observation of procedural due process safeguards during the commitment process.

Starting with the case of *Heryford* v. *Parker* in 1968,* courts have emphasized new rights in the commitment process designed to make it more difficult to put a patient into a state mental hospital and to retain him in the hospital. *Heryford* v. *Parker* is a federal case involving the continued holding of a mentally retarded man under the terms of a Wyoming statute which provided that the proposed patient "may be represented by counsel." The case stands for the proposition that there is not an optional but an obligatory right to counsel at each state of the proceedings even when, as in this case, the original commitment had been of a minor and his parents had waived the right to counsel. The reason for this—the case stands for this important proposition in this jurisdiction and in others where it has been cited as authority—is that the court sees no real difference between the loss of liberty caused by civil commitment and the loss of liberty that results from a criminal prosecution.

Beginning with this case courts have been increasingly willing to equate the benign, well-intentioned psychiatrist—or so he seems to himself—with the malevolent and punitive jailer, at least so far as the effects are on the detained individual. We thus have the rationale for a new emphasis on procedural rights. The case which had often been cited previously to justify the detention of the mentally disabled, in the *Matter of Josiah Oakes*,[11] has been explicit that dangerousness was the rationale for involuntary detention ("whether a patient's own safety, or that of others, requires that he should be restrained for a certain time") but it gave the doctors much latitude in defining dangerousness. Now the courts are tightening up the criteria. Many of the new cases analogized the plight of the patient in an involuntary commitment proceeding to the juvenile delinquent; they are both facing the loss of liberty for a therapeutic, not a punitive, purpose. The courts have said that the

*Heryford* v. *Parker*, 396 F.2d 393 (10th Cir. 1968).

same kind of minimum due process protections must be given to mental
patients that the Supreme Court said in *In re Gault** must be made
available to juveniles—the right to be represented by counsel, to be
notified of the charges which have been made, to confront and cross-
examine witnesses, to remain silent if cooperating might lead to incrim-
ination. The *Gault* case also provided that juveniles being sentenced
must have an opportunity for a review of the decision on appeal and
that an adequate record must be kept by the courts and made available
to the juvenile for that purpose.

Although courts may not feel that all the *Gault* case rights are
appropriate for the commitment proceeding, they do feel that the
principle that at least some basic rights must be afforded does apply—
and, following up on this, courts in several jurisdictions have outlawed
the medical commitment since these rights cannot be observed except
when a commitment is conducted more formally.† A number of other
jurisdictions have rewritten their commitment laws so that patients are
given more protection. Pennsylvania, Wisconsin, Alabama, Tennessee,
South Dakota, and West Virginia are all states in which courts have
recently made commitment more legally protected; California, Massachusetts, North Carolina, Virginia, and Florida are examples of states
where legislatures have emphasized that such factors as overt expressions of dangerousness, a high likelihood of dangerousness, the indication that all less restrictive alternatives have been explored, and a
continuing necessity of commitment must be shown to justify commitment or extension of the commitment.‡ A Minnesota case settled by
stipulation gives patients procedural rights when the hospital decides
either to revoke or to extend provisional discharges from the hospital;
an independent hearing examiner must be available, and contested
cases require prehearing discovery (including the right to examine
hospital records), the right to be informed of all allegations relating to
the basis for the recommended extension or revocation, the right to
witness lists, the right to cross-examine and subpoena witnesses, the
right to evidentiary safeguards at the hearings, and the requirement of

---

*In re Gault*, 387 U.S. 1 (1967).
†*Dixon* v. *Attorney General*, 325 F. Supp. 966 (M.D. Pa. 1971); *Lessard* v. *Schmidt*, 349 F.
   Supp. 1078 (E.D. Wis. 1974), *vacated* 414 U.S. 473 (1974), and 379 F. Supp. 1376 (E.D.
   Wis. 1974); *Lynch* v. *Baxley*, 43 U.S.L.W. 1102 (M.D. Ala. Dec. 14, 1974) (three judge
   court); *In re Martin*, (S.D. Bd. of Mental Illness, Pennington County, January 1974) cited
   in *Clearinghouse Review, 7* (March 1974), p. 689.
‡Lanterman-Petris-Short Act, California Welfare and Institutions Code, § 500 et seq.
   (1969); Code of Virginia § 37.1-67.1; North Carolina Laws § 122-58.1; Florida Statutes
   Annotated § 394.463; Annotated Laws of Massachusetts c. 123 § 8.

written findings of fact and conclusions of law that can facilitate an appeal of the decision.*

The Wisconsin District Court in the case of *Lessard* v. *Schmidt*† came out most forcibly for great legal protection for patients in the involuntary commitment process. The court in *Lessard* found that the civil deprivations accompanying commitment may be greater than those which go with a criminal conviction. It cites the Thomas Eagleton affair for the proposition that the stigma of hospitalization will produce difficulties for the committed individual in attempting to adjust to life outside the institution following release. Bruce Ennis, a lawyer who has been active in the right-to-treatment movement, is quoted for the proposition that "former mental patients do not get jobs" and that in the job market "it is better to be an ex-felon than an ex-patient."

The *Lessard* court goes on to make even graver charges against psychiatry. (The court's use of statistics might well be questioned; the general health and the age characteristics differ remarkably in the general population from the patient population, but the court makes only a passing mention of this.)

> Perhaps the most serious possible effect of a decision to commit an individual lies in the statistics which indicate that an individual committed to a mental institution has a much greater chance of dying than if he were left at large. Data compiled in 1966 indicate that while the death rate per 1000 persons in the general population in the United States each year is only 9.5, the rate among resident mental patients is 91.8.

The court raises the question of the propriety of commitment for conditions which may be untreatable; long-term paranoid schizophrenia, the condition diagnosed in the plaintiff in this case, is given as an example. The court emphasizes strict adherence to high standards of proof of dangerousness, but this must be proved by the criminal standard—beyond a reasonable doubt, rather than the civil standard— by the preponderance of the evidence, and the dangerousness must be based upon a finding of a recent overt act, or an attempt or threat to do substantial harm either to another or to the self. The court also holds that basic fairness requires that persons detained for civil commitment proceedings be given notice of fact that their statements to psychiatrists may tend to "incriminate them" (a term borrowed from criminal justice) in the eyes of psychiatrists and of the finder of fact in the commitment proceeding. The point raised by the *Lessard* court concerning the standard to be used to prove committability and requiring a criminal

---

*Anderson* v. *Likins*, No. 4-72-Civ.-422 (D. Minn. March 8, 1974) settled by stipulations reported in *Clearinghouse Review*, June 1974, p. 118.
†*Lessard* v. *Schmidt*.

law standard, beyond a reasonable doubt, is also beginning to be emphasized by courts in other jurisdictions. In a District of Columbia case the court ruled that in a civil commitment proof of both mental illness and dangerousness must be established by the stricter test, pointing out that the patient had never been convicted of a crime and that he had a great deal to lose by the commitment—his liberty.*

One answer that psychiatry has to the legal insistence on a more safeguarded commitment procedure is to utilize voluntary hospitalization more. The term *voluntary commitment* sounds like a misnomer and the term *voluntary admission* would seem to be more appropriate, but by usage voluntary admission is reserved for that type of entry into a mental hospital which allows a patient to leave at will without any formalities. Since most voluntary procedures entitle the hospital to retain the patient after his notice of desire to be discharged and the hospital can use the period of time to secure an involuntary commitment, or even use the threat of using the period of time to secure an involuntary commitment as the means of pressuring the patient to withdraw his request to leave, the element of coercion does remain; nevertheless these so-called voluntary procedures are favored by most psychiatrists.

Whether there is a real distinction between voluntary and involuntary hospitalization is an important question. If there is a real distinction, it would be reasonable to assume that only involuntary patients are entitled to the right to treatment; voluntary patients if they do not like the care they receive can "take their business elsewhere." Most commentators and courts dealing with the issue of right to treatment have not dealt with this question; they seem to assume, without any explicit basis, that all patients in mental hospitals would be benefited by the enforcement of the right. The literature does not seem to contain any suggestion that the right to treatment should only be applied to those wards of state hospitals which contain involuntary patients. There is the implication here that the needs of voluntary and involuntary patients are similar. If there is a difference, we can deny hospital admission to voluntary patients or provide them with a lesser standard of care. If there is no difference, then the question of the deprivation of liberty associated with involuntary commitment becomes a minor issue, not worth the attention that courts have given it in recent years. This is because we could no longer assert that the deprivation of liberty which is inflicted upon involuntary patients is the *quid pro quo* which entitles them to certain standards of care designed to restore them at the

---

*In re Ballay, 482 F.2d 648 (D.C. Cir. 1973).

earliest possible time since voluntary patients who are not deprived of their liberty are indistinguishable and deserve the same standard of care although their quid is lacking, i.e., they have not suffered a deprivation.

David Wexler, writing in the *California Law Review* on the right of patients to refuse various kinds of therapy, is anxious to point out that his right of refusal should belong as much to voluntary as to involuntary patients, and he bases this on the recognition which he says it is important that we make at the outset, "that the distinctions between voluntary and involuntary hospitalization and treatment are often murky."[12]

> Many hospital admissions technically designated as voluntary actually involve substantial elements of coercion. Gilboy and Schmidt described the process of voluntary admission to Illinois hospitals as one in which the majority of voluntary admittees entered "voluntarily" only under the threat of involuntary commitment. James Ellis' article . . . shows that although commitments of minor children by parents are legally designated as "voluntary," the children concerned may often regard the process as compulsory. Indeed, even adults, found to be mentally imcompetent or gravely disabled, may be signed into mental institutions and comparable facilities by their guardians or conservators pursuant to a process deemed "voluntary." As commitment itself falls into disfavor and becomes, by statute and case law, increasingly difficult to effectuate, the conservatorship route to mental hospital admission will probably increase markedly in popularity.

*Psychiatric Viewpoint,* a surveying service, in a 1973 questionnaire to psychiatrists, noted that it has been proposed that "voluntary" psychiatric hospitalization represents a paradox and a contradiction in terms.

> Most patients requiring hospitalization are psychotic and demonstrate disorders in reality testing. Yet, by signing a voluntary admission form, these patients make a major decision concerning their lives despite their probable mental incompetence. Moreover, once these patients are admitted, either voluntarily or involuntarily, an evaluation of their psychiatric status may lead to involuntary retention for their own safety or that of society. As such, a "voluntary hospitalization" may, in effect, be an agreement to an "involuntary hospitalization."[13]

Psychiatrists responding to this survey voted by more than 90% that "voluntary hospitalization" is a reasonable concept which should be promoted and utilized where possible, and that the mental health concepts of shorter hospitalizations, the greater use of partial hospitalization, and the building of inpatient services in local communities should be supported. Over 88% of the respondents agreed that there should be in their local communities mental health centers with no intake restrictions on diagnostic category. So many psychiatrists—

although perhaps primarily those who are in private practice and do not have the responsibility for managing state hospital patients—are sympathetic to the movement to divert support from the state hospital system and use it for community care and they also support more flexible, if not necessarily more legalistic, commitment practices.

But psychiatrists responding to this survey reveal an ambivalence concerning involuntary commitment; although by a ratio of 9:1 they felt the concept of voluntary hospitalization should be promoted and utilized where possible, by an almost equally lopsided ratio they voted in favor of involuntary hospitalization. As long as involuntary hospitalization is retained, the voluntariness of voluntary hospitalization will remain suspect.

The right-to-treatment concept has already influenced mental hospitals to admit fewer patients and to discharge more patients so that the retained patients can have a higher standard of care. Does it give the hospital the right to refuse admission or influence hospitals to refuse admission to voluntary patients or to provide them with less care in the hospital? None of the right-to-treatment cases has dealt with these basic questions.

In spite of the confusions that have been stirred up, it can be said with certainty that the conjunction of these three mental hospital reforms in the last decades—more protected commitment, the right to treatment, and community mental health—has led to recently expressed fears that state hospital services are being denied to some who need them, that many patients who should be closely followed by community services have become lost.

Two sensational cases have particularly helped focus attention on our new policy of restrictions on state hospitalization, the Sheila Broughel case and the Edmund Kemper case. Sheila Broughel was a bright but mentally disturbed 26-year-old Vassar college graduate and former *New Yorker* magazine secretary who had many experiences with psychiatrists and hospitals and had developed a deep distrust of them. She came to Washington in late January 1973 because she wanted to see "leaders" about conditions in mental hospitals. She spent the last week of her life living in Washington's seamy Union Station. She spent most of her time standing in the same spot at the entrance, even at night and in the rain. Who or what she was waiting for she would not say.

Paul Hodge, a reporter for the *Washington Post*, became concerned about her. He was at the station covering another story, discussed her with a station policeman who told him she was "crazy" but that there was nothing he could do since she was not a danger to herself or others. Hodge bought her lunch—she said she was hungry and broke—and persuaded her to go with him to see a psychiatrist he knew at St. Elizabeth's Hospital.

The psychiatrist thought she needed help and advised her to sign herself into the hospital voluntarily. She refused and asked to be taken back home—the "home" being Union Station. The reporter left her there. The next day she disappeared. Writes Hodge, "When her mutilated body, sexually assaulted and stabbed almost 30 times, was found in an abandoned garage a dozen blocks from Union Station, some of her friends and even a relative said they were not surprised and thought it to be a kind of suicide."[14]

Hodge quotes a New Haven lawyer whose firm had twice secured her release from Connecticut mental hospitals a few years earlier: He said lawyers in his office had discussed "how would we feel if something like this happened. Suppose she ends up in an alley we said. . . . Still, I think we made the right decision in working to keep her out of hospitals. She was not dangerous and she passionately wanted to be free. That's what it means to have a free society, not to lock people up all the time."

Her mother in a telephone interview gave a different point of view: "If you look at the laws you'll know the problems we had . . . under the laws no one can help anyone else."

Edmund Emil Kemper III is a 6-foot-9-inch, 280-pound Californian who had killed his grandparents when he was 15, was in the custody of juvenile authorities and then in the state mental hospital system at Atascadero State Hospital for the criminally insane until he was 21, when he was released. Three years later, on the day his psychiatric "parole" was lifted and he had been officially certified as "sane," he killed his mother and her friend; he admitted to the police that in the three-year period he had been out of institutions he had been responsible for the rape/murder/mutilations of six hitchhiking coeds.[15]

A rapidly developing literature documents the plight of the mentally ill who have been denied access to hospitals, allowed to elect to stay out of hospitals, been forced out of hospitals, or have been seen as too "well" to be kept in hospitals.

Darold Treffert, director of the Mental Health Institute of Winnebago, Winconsin, has said, "In our zeal to protect basic, human freedoms, we have created a legal climate in which mentally ill patients, and sometimes the people around them, are dying with their rights on."[16] He cites the danger to the individual and gives examples of suicides and a death from anorexia nervosa, the danger to others from an out-of-control mentally ill person, and also the destruction of family life:

Sometimes the family of a psychotic mother may literally disintegrate while vainly trying to construct some form of routine family life around mother's bizarre and often psychologically destructive symptoms. Or the wife of a mentally ill man may finally abandon her struggle to keep the family going, wearied by fruitless attempts to patch together the semblance of a normal marriage.

A recent issue of *Psychiatric Annals* with the theme "Psychiatry Under Siege" contains the Reich and Siegel article with the arresting title, "The Chronically Mentally Ill Shuffle to Oblivion." It describes the reaction in New York to a 1968 memo from the Department of Mental Hygiene stating it was the duty of state hospital directors to ascertain in the case of every patient and especially in the case of elderly patients that state hospital care is the most appropriate treatment:

> Word got around quickly to municipal and voluntary hospitals that the state hospital system was, by and large, only accepting the acutely mentally ill. To protect themselves from clogging acute general hospital psychiatric beds with chronic cases, the general hospitals as well began to refuse admission to the chronically ill, who were turned back to the community. Many of these patients had no families or were too disturbed for normal family living, and so the welfare system had to find places for these sick people to live.
>
> The "new policy" has taxed to the limit already overburdened facilities in the community. Tremendous hardship has been sustained by the families of discharged patients and, where families do not exist, by the community in general. Many incidents of physical violence have occurred. In the streets, of course, the problem is more profound and widespread. Alcoholics further deteriorate; young schizophrenics are deprived of their only chance for some guidance, support and treatment; and recluses are not even thought of—because they don't bother anyone and do not ask for help. Patients are lost to follow-up, discontinue medications, and in deteriorated condition sleep in the streets or the subways. They often cannot care for their own needs and frequently pose a threat to themselves or others. The age of phenothiazines and liberalized psychiatric thinking has released patients from their strait jackets and back wards into the oblivion and slow desperation of furnished rooms, run-down hotels and subway station domiciles.[17]

The problem of the homeless mentally disabled is with us, and legal pressure continues for still further reductions in hospital populations. A paper presented at the Canadian Psychiatric Association states:

> If . . . large numbers of patients discharged from mental hospitals have joined the ranks of the homeless and prison populations, the radical changes in management of severe psychiatric syndromes in western countries during the last decade may prove to have had a less satisfactory impact upon patient status than commonly supposed.[18]

One problem with policies of maintaining psychiatric patients outside of hospitals is that communities often do not want them, and exclusionary tactics—both ordinances that prohibit them from geographical areas and administrative policies that foster "ghettoization"—may relegate the mentally ill, in the words of one article, "to the back alleys" of the community.[19]

There are beginning to be some second thoughts. California, which had announced plans to phase out its state mental hospitals by 1982, now plans to keep state institutions going for the "foreseeable future."[20]

Janet Chase states in a *Human Behavior* article[21] that since 1969, the date of California's more restrictive commitment act, there have been at least 72 cases of murders, suicides, and "unfortunate accidents" that have directly involved either former patients or people for whom psychiatric care could not be obtained. A man released from Camarillo State Hospital after observation because he did not meet the criteria for commitability—violent behavior in the three-day observation period—two weeks later killed his wife, three of his five children, and himself. Another man being released from an honor camp told an officer, "I don't want to go out there. I feel like a puppy you're putting on the freeway. I don't think I can make it." A number of years later he was charged with committing—in a two-day, 500-mile chase—two murders, two rapes, the kidnapping of several families, and the assault of two police officers; he is suspected of being a rapist and killer of Asian women around San Francisco's Chinatown.

A preamble to the Chase article reads:

> In 1969, California's bill of rights for the mentally ill was widely hailed as a piece of liberal legislation that would benefit both patient and society. After all, who would argue against liberating patients from the snake pits where many were kept against their will? But once the asylum doors opened, there were some unwelcome and unforeseen happenings. Obviously something is going wrong, and the time has come for a serious reappraisal.

Most of the California patients were not dangerous to others, but many of them were not capable of taking care of themselves and so from a psychiatric viewpoint, but possibly not a legal viewpoint, could be seen as dangerous, or at least as damaging to themselves. (It is often pointed out by critics of state hospitals that studies of released mental patients, including the 969 end-of-sentence, "criminally insane" men that as a result of the court order in the *Baxstrom* case* were transferred from New York's Dannemora and Matteawan State Hospitals although psychiatrists had testified they were too dangerous to be moved, show they are no more dangerous and may be less dangerous than matched groups.[22] The fallacy here is that no studies exist on patients who are recently ill or floridly ill. Many of the patients included in the studies

---

*Baxtrom* v. *Herold*, 383 U.S. 107 (1966).

which disprove dangerousness deal with former mental patients, discharged after long periods of hospitalization as sufficiently improved to live in the community, or with end-of-sentence prisoners who have been retained in mental hospitals; these are often chronic patients in an older age group who would not be expected to show the capacity for unpredictable behavior and for aggressive and violent acting out that may be seen in a younger and more acute patient.)

Many released California patients end up in board-and-care homes, a term that applies both to family dwellings housing under six patients and to renovated motels and licensed convalescent hospitals that house 100 or more. Here entrepreneurs sell services that traditionally have been provided by the state or by charitable organizations on a not-for-profit basis. Chase reports that the quality of these facilities varies widely; some have doctors on call, recreational therapy, transportation to mental health centers; others are "old, rundown buildings that can meet no fire or other safety requirements, have no medical personnel on hand and house mentally ill, retarded and alcoholics of both sexes together." State mental health officials are quoted as saying that conditions in most board-and-care homes are "splendid." State Senator Alfred Alquist says conditions are "deplorable."

The article describes the springing up of convalescent hospitals since California started to reduce its inpatient population; one chain is owned by a company called Beverly Enterprises, which started out with three convalescent facilities in 1964 and today owns 63 board-and-care facilities and 12 general hospitals, and has additional land holdings. In 1971 its revenue was $67 million; in 1972 this had increased to $79 million.

This then is another possible reason for the attempted phaseout of state mental hospitals; the entrepreneurs who run nursing homes see a possibility of expanding their efforts in the field of mental patient care. Reformers who are attempting to close mental hospitals must ask themselves if they are the agents of a new kind of mental patient exploitation. It should be noted that the announced phaseout of the California state mental hospital systems has been variously described as a progressive and humanistic reform and as a regressive measure by then Governor Reagan to aid the financial fortunes of the private mental health care industry.

Studies in California and New York show that a great amount of consistent community care is needed if a large percentage of former state hospital patients are to be maintained in the community. But continuity of care is not available in many community mental health centers, which are themselves sometimes chaotic and disorganized.

Community clinics have personnel problems; they often have a high rate of personnel turnover, a great reliance on workers without professional training, the de-emphasis of the more highly trained professional (who is often used merely to endorse the recommendations of workers who do not have the status or authority to be responsible for admissions, discharges, and medication orders), and wide fluctuations in financing which lead to staff discontinuity. They often lack a unified treatment philosophy, and patients get a touch of social work, a little chemotherapy, a little directive therapy, and rarely any insight therapy—all provided by a multiplicity of therapists and workers. The main characteristic of good patient care—a strong and continued interest in the welfare of one individual (the patient) by another (the therapist)—is usually lacking. And the costs of this kind of care are, in the description of Dr. Robert Gibson, "astronomical."[23] The cost in the community mental health center may be over $100 per patient visit, which visit may be merely for gathering of information, a brief follow-up, or in other ways less than a real and lengthy therapeutic contact. Studies of clinic practice show that much time of personnel goes to continuing education, staff conferences, organizational and administrative work; the patient is not the sole concern—perhaps not even the primary object—of the community mental health center. The maintenance of the organization becomes a focus of concern.

Under these circumstances, it is fanciful to think that a discharged hospital patient will necessarily find a worker in the community who can relate to him in an important and stable fashion. A California study indicates that releasing patients earlier means that many more are available to come back than before. Dorothy Miller writes:

> We have found in our study of 1,405 California patients on leave of absence that what allows a mental patient to stay out is not primarily the severity of his medical diagnosis and prognosis. It depends on whether he has been able to (or has been helped to) construct a social and psychological world that will support him and allow him to function adequately in the outside world.[24]

Although Miller's study described patients who were released in the 1950s and thus had been subject to longer term hospitalizations than today's patients with more disruption of family and community ties, the description of the patients sounds suspiciously like many of today's released patients. The rate of marriage in the patient population was only 56% of the rate in the general adult population. The majority of former mental patients had only marginal or casual connections with their families. They were not heads of homes, they were not important in family maintenance and support. They were often "unwelcome guests in other people's homes. . . . Generally they were important to nobody." After discharge only 16% could find any kind of full-time job, and another 16% found "sheltered" or part-time jobs.

Many lived alone, typically in skid row hotels, and were on relief. Others lived with parents who were frequently aged and infirm. Says Miller, "These mental patients lived in, or with, the kinds of families that make up the hard core of social case work, disrupted, problem-ridden, often apparently hopeless. Their mental and domestic troubles were inseparable, being so closely intertwined that cause and effect were seldom clear. Often their return to the mental hospital was just one more result of social and family disruption."

The California experience has been paralleled in other parts of the country. The *New York Times,* after a continuing investgation, concluded that thousands of released mental patients are getting little or no treatment; it quoted officials of the American Psychiatric Association as saying that programs for released mental patients were working poorly. It gave as an example the release to New York City for placement of a group of fifty patients from Willowbrook, an institution for the retarded. The city found about half of the fifty unfit for community living and returned them to Willowbrook. The rest were placed in nursing homes for the elderly which lacked special programs for the retarded. The private nursing homes were "health-related facilities," which means that they had little medical care. The elderly are often terrified when retardates and former mental patients are placed in their facility. Retardates in other states have been released to "skilled nursing facilities" where more medical care is available—although the retarded usually do not need this kind of care—but where the other special needs of the retarded are overlooked.[25]

In the early 1960s an experiment was designed to determine whether acute psychotics could be treated in their homes rather than in state mental hospitals. The initial findings were that the home-care patients did better than the hospital patients; such studies gave impetus to the community-care movement. A follow-up study on the same patients from 1962 to 1969 showed that the home-care group was no longer significantly different from the hospital group and both groups had continued to deteriorate. The study concluded that close and continuing supervision with the maintenance of drug therapy is needed to minimize and prevent recurrent psychotic episodes. These chronic patients are the patients that community mental health has neglected. They do not take their medicine, they do not seek help, they do not show up for appointments, they are lost in the anonymity of the community.[26]

More recent studies give similar conclusions. Reibel and Herz, in a group of 112 carefully selected patients, found brief hospitalization combined with a follow-up program of living at home and hospital day care was not sufficient for 9 out of their 112 patients.[27] The relatively new ideology of brief hospitalization and rapid return to the community "is not categorically effective or humane," they say. A wholesale acceptance of the policy can place "intolerable burdens upon individual patients, their families and society."

They conclude that there is no simple answer to the question of who should leave and who should stay in the hospital. "Family, social, and individual factors seemed to be combined in a rather subtle and often elusive fashion to create a situation which was not remediable by means of brief hospital care, with or without transitional day care." They give as factors which are involved in failure: homicidal and suicidal ideation or behavior, family-related problems such as disorganization, and treatment failure; less often reported are psychotic disorganization, antisocial behavior, and mental deficiency leading to poor judgment or impulsive behavior.

The question is not whether state mental hospitals have needed to be improved; they have been deficient and investigators have been able to document stories of neglected, misdiagnosed, undertreated, and overcontrolled patients who have been retained in hospitals too long. They have been underfinanced, they have usually been custodially oriented rather than therapy-oriented, and they have lacked support and input from the main body of American psychiatrists who practice private psychiatry without contact with or relationship to the state mental hospital. The state hospital as it has existed would find few defenders. The question is whether court-imposed policies—to allow hospitalization only when there is current overt dangerousness, to impose on state hospitals standards which must be obeyed at the risk of a citation for contempt of court, to determine the social policy of forcing patients to be treated in the community whether or not the community is ready to treat them—will secure better patient care. And while the battle has been waged in the courts, organized psychiatry has been relieved of the responsibility of being the architect and agent of hospital improvement; it has sat back and waited for court directives instead of undertaking the task itself.

In 1967 Dr. Lewis Bartlett pinpointed some of the main deficiencies in the state hospital system, and he predicted they would become worse rather than better if mental hospitals continued to be isolated from the main stream of psychiatry.[28] He felt that the indigent-welfare designation of institutionalized patients, the antiquated standards of medical staffing, and the forced labor of hospital patients guaranteed a low standard of care for patients. The right-to-treatment cases have attempted to deal with these problems, but only with the last of these— forced patient labor or institutional peonage, which it prohibited—has it been successful.

Patients have been prohibited by the *Wyatt* case order to perform hospital labor unless that labor is either voluntary and paid for in accordance with minimum wages set by the Fair Labor Standards Act or is an integrated part of the patient's treatment plan and does not involve the maintenance and operation of the hospital. A case with application to all jurisdictions that similarly requires patients to be paid for the work that maintains institutions is *Souder* v. *Brennan*,* which orders the secretary of labor to apply the Fair Labor Standards Act to patient labor. Comments *Behavior Today*: "One of the many ironies of the patient pay issue is that with a few exceptions, the only mental institutions in full, safe compliance with anti-peonage laws right now are those that have phased out resident work."[29]

The state hospital patient will continue to be treated like an indigent as long as he is not entitled to the same financial support for his hospitalization that the private mental patient receives; the disparity of care in the two-tier mental health system is largely the result of health insurance plans that do little for most mentally ill. The special licensing of otherwise ineligible physicians continues to be a main source—in most states *the* main source—of hospital medical staff; doctors working on institutional rather than regular state licenses treat patients even though they may have had no psychiatric training and may not have good command of English.

Bartlett quotes an editorial in the *New England Journal of Medicine* entitled "He That Was Dead, Came Forth": "Perhaps it is too often believed that miracles are required in psychiatry, when very often simple mortal acts will get the job done."[28] The deficiencies which Bartlett describes do not require detailed court orders, the usurpation of psychiatric authority by judges and lawyers, the imposition of judicial control over the legislative appropriation function; they require some broad legal injunctions such as Birnbaum originally described to ensure that public care is not below the standard for private care and they demand the concern of responsible psychiatrists.

The "simple mortal acts"—which should not require court action for their exercise—will not be performed as long as state hospital psychiatry is as unimportant as it is to most of psychiatry. As Bartlett wrote in another paper, "In this century . . . the state hospital superin-

*Souder* v. *Brennan*, 367 F. Supp. 808 (D.D.C. 1973).

tendents, their hospitals and their staffs have continued to suffer a kind of downgrading and have lost the status associated with the mid-19th century state hospitals. . . . [T]he state hospitals and their essential services seem to be in the position of being wished away."[30] He pointed out that state hospital superintendents in most of this century have not had a compelling voice in American psychiatry; they have not had major input into the formulation of the community mental health center scheme; if they had, this plan would have been tailored more to the needs of the state hospital patient and less to the social and political needs of the average man. Bartlett's call was for the state mental hospital to join the community.

We have now had a chance to evaluate the effect of the right-to-treatment concept as set forth in the *Wyatt* case regulations on Alabama hospital patients, and although no studies have emerged, newspaper accounts tell us of the continued problems that plague Alabama in spite of the court-ordered right. The fate of Dr. Stonewall Stickney, the state mental health commissioner for Alabama who was the ostensible defendant in the suit but who had actually welcomed it because he wanted legal pressure to help him in his fight to improve patient care, is particularly instructive. Before the suit was instituted, Stickney's program for Alabama had included such progressive goals as the decentralization of mental health treatment, the building of regional mental health centers, and the reduction of the population of hospitals by returning to private homes those patients who were simply in need of custodial care or geriatric nursing.

After the court had enunciated the doctrine of a constitutionally guaranteed right to treatment, had given the state an opportunity to improve its services, and had expressed its disapproval of the lack of improvements, Stickney and his codefendants proposed conditions they considered compatible with a minimal treatment program, but these stipulations were entered into at a time of pressure and represent a bargain from a position of weakness on the part of the defendants. The patient–personnel ratio of 250:207.5 seems particularly hard to justify.

But acceding to the pressure from the court and conceding all rights did not relieve Stickney of the pressure from his legislature and his mental health board, and as a result of *Wyatt*, he was fired. Previously he had fired his deputy commissioner, Dr. James Folsom. The next commissioner of mental health for Alabama was not a doctor, he was the department's finance officer. The transition from a system dominated by physicians to a system dominated by accountants has great significance: It is part of a nationwide pattern of subordinating the role of the psychiatrist, emphasizing administrators and financial experts, and of putting psychiatry on a costs–benefits basis. At the time accountant Charles Aderholt took the job, one mental health board member made the comment, "Well, we've got a new pitcher, we're still ten runs behind and it's the last inning of this ball game." Aderholt lasted a year. When he resigned, his post went to another nonphysician, a member of Governor Wallace's cabinet, State Finance Director Taylor Hardin.[31]

Changes have been wrought in the system, but these changes were generally initiated by Stickney before the suit was brought. By moving patients out and by limiting admissions, the state has cut the population of its mental institutions from in excess of 10,000 to less than 6,000: Spending in the institutions has gone from $14 million yearly to $54 million;[32] cost per patient per day has gone from $6.86 (with only $.50 representing the cost of food) to $17.25 and is projected to rise to $25.00. But the manpower requirements which Judge Johnson mandated as constitutional minimums are not being met. A follow-up report on the effects of the order in the *Wall Street Journal* stated that Bryce and Searcy Hospitals, which should have had a total of 52 licensed physicians, still had only 13.[33] (The newspaper was not quite correct; the terms of the court order—2 psychiatrists and 4 other physicians for every 250 patients—would require not 52 but 96 licensed physicians for the nearly 4,000 patients in Bryce and Searcy.) Partlow State School and Hospital for the mentally retarded still had only 3 doctors; their average age was 66 and the eldest was 78. One had cataracts and the other 2 had had strokes.

The manpower shortage at the three institutions has continued in spite of the increased funding and the court order. Finally *Psychiatric News*, the official paper of the American Psychiatric Association, was impelled into action. After a classified advertisement had appeared in the back of the newspaper for many months and had not had any response, it was reproduced as part of an editorial entitled "Unanswered."[34] The advertisement said there were immediate openings for five board-certified or board-eligible psychiatrists at Bryce Hospital (actually, there should have been openings for many more psychiatrists to comply with the court-ordered patient–staff ratio). Salaries were negotiable upward from $33,371 for board-eligible and $36,792 for board-certified psychiatrists.

The editorial called attention to Judge Johnson's order, which it described as containing enough specifics "to fill a volume, ranging from staff-to-patient ratios to the frequency of linen changes." It said that Bryce was being looked at throughout the country by civil liberties groups and the judiciary because the *Wyatt* case has become "a watershed of patients' rights." It pleaded with psychiatrists—not only ordinary run-of-the-mill psychiatrists but even older psychiatrists in retirement or younger psychiatrists who would altruistically spend a limited period of time in this service even though they did not want to seek a long-term career in the state hospital system—to answer the advertisement.

The absence of any follow-up story to this unusual editorial/advertisement leads to the conclusions that "Unanswered" too has probably gone unanswered. Court decrees do not solve manpower problems as long as physicians have the freedom to pick their places of employment. (It can be noted that Dr. Thomas Szasz, who takes an extreme civil libertarian point of view on every issue, has attacked the right to treatment for patients as carrying with it the physicians' obligation to treat, which could lead to interference with the freedom of doctors to practice under conditions of their own choosing.)

The increased expenditures at Bryce have not earned high praise for the hospital. One result has been the adoption of *ersatz* therapeutic modalities which would not be recognized in private hospitals. One expert who visited Bryce said that not only was there a "frightful shortage of mental health professionals," but that "the staff interviewed, with few exceptions, reflected no awareness of what might constitute a therapeutic experience for patients." One patient who ran errands for the hospital staff was rewarded with points which could be used to buy canteen items; the staff described this as a behavior modification program, but the visiting expert stated, "A more gross distortion of behavior-modification therapy can hardly be conjured up."[33]

The court has imposed its own behavior modification scheme, which is also a gross distortion of behavior modification therapy, on the hospital. Under the threat of punishment the hospital must "comply"; its compliance does not necessarily indicate any thoughtful or useful change of direction for the hospital but merely a hasty attempt to deflect the wrath of the court. The result is the elevation of low-cost but unproven treatment modalities, even those used in watered-down versions, to the status of that treatment to which the patient has a right.

Governor Wallace has recently, perhaps exaggeratedly, estimated that it would cost the state of Alabama $110 million to provide the air conditioning, patient space requirements, personnel, and all the other requirements contained in the pages of orders that the courts have imposed on the hospital system. That price would not be high if good patient care resulted, but the court order which emphasizes all other phases of patient treatment, to the point of specifying how many chaplains, messengers, dieticians, and maintenance repairmen are needed for every unit of patients, does not deal with the question of how much and what kind of therapy should be provided. Providing the most cost-effective treatment will mean that factors other than kind and quality of care will be the criteria of the new finance officer-hospital system head; and reward schemes known euphemistically as behavior modification, chemotherapy, and electroshock can be expected to be the treatment modalities most employed when the right to treatment is fully implemented. This will be no worse than the treatment state hospital patients have traditionally received, but now physicians can view this with good conscience, because they are in conformance with court orders, instead of seeing this as a situation in need of change.

Dr. Seymour Halleck, a thoughtful and liberal psychiatrist who has wanted other psychiatrists to be more conscious of social forces, has written of the demands that the new court-directed psychiatry makes on the psychiatrist. The psychiatrist can now spend more and more time in court debates, or merely waiting for the debate to begin, at the expense of his time as a healer. "If the psychiatrist goes to court as often as the new laws requires, the psychiatrist's effectiveness as a healer will diminish. . . . [T]he situation will improve only if we train many more psychiatrists or find some legal means of making the psychiatrist's appearance in court as brief as possible."[35]

He adds that "the value of 'personal liberty' is taking precedence over the value of 'mental health.' . . . It is possible . . . that if we continue to value liberty so exclusively we may at some point in the future find ourselves in an antihumanistic position. . . .

"There have undoubtedly been atrocities committed against the mentally ill," he writes, "as a result of insufficient protection of their legal rights. But these atrocities pale in comparison to the harm done to the mentally ill by failing to provide them with the treatment they might need."

Dr. Russell Barton, director of the Rochester, New York, Psychiatric Center, has said, "A mental hospital, if properly run, does serve a purpose. It gives a haven and a security. We have no right to abandon people until we have alternative facilities."[36]

Dr. Philip May, professor of psychiatry at the University of California, Los Angeles, has proposed that the old psychiatric hospital could be turned into a core unit-of-care with responsibility for and cooperation with satellite community outpatient facilities. There could be easy flow back and forth between the satellites and the sponsoring institutions. Such a scheme would counter the present deficiencies of the community mental health centers which overlook chronic psychotic patients in their efforts to treat patients in the general population who have not needed hospitalization and who fail to keep up continuity of care and active supervision of discharged hospital patients.[36]

State mental hospitals can serve a purpose, and they are capable of reformation from inside of psychiatry. Court-imposed reforms will not work because courts see the problems of hospitals as simpler and more capable of change by edict than they are in actuality. Lawyers and judges, not having the responsibility for patient care, plan the ideal therapeutic situation while doctors, responsible for the protection of patients and of society, find it difficult to implement these ideal plans. Lawyers and judges do not conceptualize the mentally disabled as irrational, but merely as unfortunate. They impose reforms that are not in harmony with any potential for growth and development which the state hospital system may still possess.

Courts have not found answers to the problems of the criminal justice system, to the mistreatment of prisoners, to disparity of sentencing, to the squalid conditions of youth detention centers, to court delays and inefficiencies and financial extravagances; until courts have shown skill in ordering the house of justice it seems arrogant for them to dictate to the reordering of mental health care. And court intervention deep into the internal administration of state hospitals represents an invasion of the territory of the administrative branch of the government where courts until very recently have refused to go because of the threat to the concept of a government with three equally powerful branches related to each other by checks and balances. The constitutional question of the power of the judiciary may in future years turn out to be the most important issue in the new legalistic approach to mental hospitalization.

Improvements in the state hospital system can come, if they come at all, only from within psychiatry. The American Psychiatric Association must recognize this as our primary psychiatric problem. University training programs must include care of state hospital patients in their teaching programs. The abdication of responsibility for the public patient by the private practitioner must be ended—perhaps by an obligation to spend some time in state hospital work as a prerequisite for eligibility to call oneself a psychiatric specialist (although this plan calls up images of the unfree physician which Szasz so much fears). The two-tier system and the use of substandard psychiatrists in the state hospital system must be ended. Private for-profit psychiatric hospitals should not be allowed to skim off the top mental health dollars. These are reforms which the courts have not begun to consider; they are the kinds of reforms that cannot be imposed from outside but must develop from an assumption of social responsibility by psychiatry, by a desire to do something better than what has been done.

The *British Medical Journal* in 1973 stated that between 1960 and 1969 British mental hospitals lost 24,000 beds in pursuance of official government policy. The mental life of Britain did not noticeably improve as a result. "There is . . . evidence enough that the run-down of our mental hospitals has contributed in an unwholesome number of cases to a life of rootless wandering in which reception centers, common lodging houses, prisons and park benches are the only available resting-places. It is hard to believe that such an existence of aimless destitution is preferable to the organized and structured life in a well-run mental hospital, even taking into account the hazards of so-called institutionalization."[37]

An American counterpart to this opinion has been expressed by Dr. Alan Stone, like Seymour Halleck one of psychiatry's liberal spokesmen who nevertheless has fears about the impact of the new legalism:

> Most psychiatrists, myself among them, believe that the new onslaught of law has cut away at the psychiatric enterprise without adequate consideration or respect for our difficult mission—the provision of mental health care. In the name of the Constitution and civil rights, serious impediments to the provision of mental health care have been erected, and the mentally ill, particularly the chronically mentally ill, have been abandoned to their rights.
>
> Many state legislatures have followed the lead of the courts and pushed through sweeping reforms of their mental health laws without providing the funds or the alternative facilities that such changes mandate if treatment is to take place.
>
> Even the so-called right-to-treatment suits have thus far resulted in the reduction of institution census rather than the improvement of quality of care. If psychiatry is to resist this assault, it must do more than grumble and cavil; it must inform itself, understand the relevant legal issues, and then provide direction to the necessary progress of law.[38]

History tells us that there have been previous ebbs and flows in the treatment of mental patients. In 1860 an English psychiatrist wrote:

> The tide of public opinion has set strongly against asylums; soon, however, it will be slack water, and then a few outrages will probably turn the prejudices of the fickle public against the liberty of mad folk. A few striking examples are sufficient to turn the direction of public opinion.[39]

Says Halleck, "If the level of chaos in our society increases to an intolerable level there is likely to be a 'conservative backlash' which will affect many of our social institutions including our system for treating the mentally disordered."[35] Rather than subject the mentally ill to extreme pushes and pulls which at one time leave them undercontrolled and at another overcontrolled, good mental health practice dictates that we do more for patients, but not in the ways which the courts are now forcing on psychiatry. By making commitment too difficult and by releasing many patients to communities where facilities are either unavailable or ineffectual, we are not helping mental patients.

The problem of the state hospital patient and the ex-hospital patient can be viewed in a broad perspective as typical of many problems of our times which have demanded change but which have not benefited from gradiose schemes of reform. Even many ardent liberals are beginning to see that their reform plans have often upset existing structures, disturbed equilibria which, as undesirable as they are, may be better than alternatives. Shana Alexander writes in a news column, "In a season of remorse, of guilt and anxiety over the mistakes of the recent past, it seems only natural to find the country swept by a panic to reform. . . . I take note of the rising pressures for no-fault divorce, no-fault insurance, no-dirt porn, and what I would call no-fault medical malpractice. Add to all this the burgeoning cries of liberal purists to clean out, or throw out, the CIA; of prison reformers to let everybody out of jail; of psychiatrists to open up the mental hospitals . . . and one can but look for comfort in Hazlitt's observation that 'it is essential to the triumph of reform that it should never succeed.'"[40]

## References

1. Szasz, T. *Law, liberty and psychiatry*. New York: Macmillan, 1963; *The manufacture of madness*. New York: Harper & Row, 1970. Dershowitz, A. The psychiatrist's power in civil commitment: A knife that cuts both ways. *Psychology Today*, February 1969, p. 43. Ennis, B., & Litwack, T. Psychiatry and the presumption of expertise: Flipping coins in the courtroom. *California Law Review*, 1974, 62 (May), pp. 693, 745; fn. 182. Ennis, B. Civil liberties and mental illness. *Criminal Law Bulletin*, 1971, 7, 101.
2. Birnbaum, M. The right to treatment. *American Bar Association Journal*, 1960, 46, 499; A new right. *American Bar Association Journal*, 1960, 46, 516; *Basic rights of the mentally handicapped*. Washington, D.C.: Mental Health Law Project, 1973.
3. Robitscher, J. The right to treatment: A social–legal approach to the plight of the state hospital patient. *Villanova Law Review*, 1972, 18, 11; Implementing the rights of the mentally disabled: Judicial, legislative and psychiatric action. In F. Ayd (Ed.), *Medical, moral and legal issues in mental health care*. Baltimore: Williams and Wilkins, 1974.
4. Birnbaum, M. The right to treatment: Some comments on its development. In F. Ayd (Ed.), *Medical, moral and legal issues in mental health care*. Baltimore: Williams and Wilkins, 1974. P. 122.
5. Birnbaum, M. The right to treatment: Some comments on its development. In F. Ayd (Ed.), *Medical, moral and legal issues in mental health care*. Baltimore: Williams and Wilkins, 1974. P. 98.

6. Pear, R. Court broadens rights of mental patients. *Washington Star,* December 29, 1975, p. 1.
7. *Mental Retardation Facilities and Community Mental Health Centers Construction Act of 1963, Public Law 88–164, 88th Congress.* Message of President John Kennedy to Congress, February 1963.
8. National Institute of Mental Health statistics, provision personnel and financial data, inpatient services of state and county medical hospitals, July 1, 1972–June 30, 1973. *Mental Health Scope,* November 20, 1974, pp. 1, 4.
9. Birnbaum, M. The right to treatment: Some comments on its development. In F. Ayd (Ed.), *Medical, moral and legal issues in mental health care.* Baltimore: Williams and Wilkins, 1974. Pp. 129–130.
10. Birnbaum, M. The right to treatment: Some comments on its development. In F. Ayd (Ed.), *Medical, moral and legal issues in mental health care.* Baltimore: Williams and Wilkins, 1974. p. 131.
11. *Matter of Josiah Oakes,* 8 Law Reporter 123 (Mass. Sup. Ct. 1845). In S. J. Brakel & R. S. Rock, *The mentally disabled and the law* (2nd ed.). Chicago: University of Chicago Press, 1971.
12. Wexler, D. Mental health law and the movement toward voluntary treatment. *California Law Review,* 1974, *62,* 671, 676.
13. Survey 1973. *Psychiatric Viewpoints,* 1974.
14. Hodge, P. Murder victim's last years were a confused call for help. *Washington Post,* March 19, 1973, p. 1.
15. Chase, J. Where have all the patients gone? *Human Behavior,* 1973, October, 14.
16. Treffert, D. Dying with their rights on. *Prism,* 1974, February, 49–52.
17. Reich, R., & Siegel, L. The chronically mentally ill shuffle to oblivion. *Psychiatric Annals,* 1973, *3*(11), 35–55.
18. Eastwood, M. R. *Risks of premature discharge.* Address to Canadian Psychiatric Association. *Psychiatric News,* August 1, 1973, p. 20.
19. Aviram, U., & Segal, S. Exclusion of the mentally ill. *Archives of General Psychiatry,* 1973, No. 29 (July), 126–131.
20. California shelves plans for abolishing hospitals. *Psychiatric News,* December 19, 1973, p. 1.
21. Chase, J. Where have all the patients gone? *Human Behavior,* 1973, October, 14–21.
22. Steadman, H., & Halfon, A. The Baxstrom patients: Background and outcomes. *Seminars in Psychiatry,* August 1971, *3,*(3) 376–385.
23. Gibson, R. *Critical issues for psychoanalysis and psychiatry in national health insurance.* Talk to the Atlanta Psychoanalytic Society, January 31, 1975.
24. Miller, D. Worlds that fail. *Trans-Action,* 1966, December, 36–41.
25. Schumach, M. U.S. casts doubt on states' mental health reviews. *New York Times,* September 29, 1974, p. 24.
26. Davis, A. E., Dinitz, S., & Pasamanick, B. The prevention of hospitalization in schizophrenia: Five years after an experimental program. *American Journal of Orthopsychiatry,* 1972, *42,* 375–388.
27. Brief hospitalization philosophy carries potent dangers, M.D.'s say. *Mental Health Scope,* June 14, 1974, p. 1.
28. Bartlett, L. Present-day requirements for state hospitals joining the community. *New England Journal of Medicine,* 1967, *276,* 90–94.
29. From peonage to pay. *Behavior Today,* January 20, 1975, p. 364.
30. Bartlett, L. *The third mental health revolution and the state hospital superintendents.* Presented at annual meeting of the Association of Medical Superintendents of Mental Hospitals, Washington, D.C., September 30, 1968.

31. Wasson, D. F. Mental health chief named after firing. *Atlanta Journal and Constitution,* October 1, 1972, p. C-2.
32. *Atlanta Journal and Constitution,* December 23, 1973, p. B-8.
33. Shils, J. Treatment, not custody: Federal court order brings big changes in lives of mentally ill and retarded patients in Alabama. *Wall Street Journal,* December 18, 1973, p. 42.
34. Unanswered. *Psychiatric News* 1974, *11*(5), 2.
35. Halleck, S. A troubled view of current trends in forensic psychiatry. *Journal of Psychiatry and Law,* 1974, Summer, 135–157.
36. Mental patients are being thrown on community. *Clinical Psychiatry News,* December 1974, p. 1.
37. Rootless wanderers. *British Medical Journal,* 1973 7 (July), 1–2.
38. Stone, A. (Reviewer). R. Slovenko, *Psychiatry and law. American Journal of Psychiatry* 1975, *132,* 89.
39. Rollin, H. My clinical hobby-horse: Talking horse sense. *World Medicine,* 1974, *13* (March), 86.
40. Alexander, S. The panic to reform. *Newsweek,* January 20, 1975, p. 84.

# 12

# Is the Community Ready?

HUGH G. LAFAVE, FREDERIC GRUNBERG,
RICHARD W. WOODHOUSE, AND LEO BARRINGTON

The myriad of mental hospitals which blight our continent should be dismantled and could be within ten years. The know-how to accomplish this has been at hand for at least as long. Institutional treatment has persisted not out of necessity but because of the interplay of an irrational ideology, misallocation of resources, ignorance of proven techniques, and local fears of the economic consequences of closing hospitals.

There is a circle of support for the existing system that includes many elements and many people: professionals in the institutions who want to perpetuate their services and their own positions; politicians and bureaucrats who accept the opinions of these professionals or who themselves have a vested interest in wanting established programs to continue within their monumental buildings; and the unsuspecting community, its families and individuals, who are told by experts time and again that institutionalization is the only way. Some people in our communities do behave in ways that others find incomprehensible or obnoxious, and without adequate services they become difficult to live

HUGH G. LAFAVE • Eleanor Roosevelt Developmental Services, Schenectady, New York 12304.    FREDERICK GRUNBERG • Albany Medical College, Union University, Schenectady, New York 12308.    RICHARD W. WOODHOUSE • Eleanor Roosevelt Developmental Services, Schenectady, New York 12304.    LEO BARRINGTON • Regis College, Weston, Massachusetts 02193.

with. Their relatives are put upon, tire of trying to cope, and are offered institutionalization as a way out.

The end product of this is the institution—a contemporary version of Plato's solution of 2,500 years ago that the disabled be abandoned to perish on a mountaintop, of the ship of fools of the 13th-century Rhineland, and of the poorhouses of more recent history. All these have been repetitious and unrealistic attempts to deal with serious and pervasive problems in the society.

One still hears voices in the 20th century claiming that mental hospitals are beneficial or a necessity. Why do some professionals continue to hold such views? At times the apologists for the mental hospital work in institutions, and have a vested interest in maintaining them.[1] At others, they work in community programs, and so are able to ignore just how bad total institutions still are.[2,3]

It appears to require a good deal of experience working in and observing both institutional and community-based systems before one gets the full sense of how terrible the best mental hospitals are, how atrocious the worst, and how readily something better can be substituted for them.

Harry Solomon, in his presidential address at the 1958 APA convention, said, "The large mental hospital is antiquated and outmoded and rapidly becoming obsolete. I do not see how any reasonably objective view of our mental hospitals today can fail to conclude that they are bankrupt and beyond remedy . . . that our large mental hospitals should be liquidated as rapidly as can be done in an orderly and progressive fashion."[4] Similar positions were taken by the American Joint Commission on Mental Illness and Health in 1961,[5] the Committee on Psychiatric Services in Canada in 1963,[6] and the Royal Commission on Health Services in Canada in 1964.[7]

And so it goes in endless procession. Fourteen years after Solomon's address, Bruce Ennis in 1972 added his name to the long list of people who have spotlighted the plight of those kept in institutions. Ennis is an activist lawyer who uses the judicial system as an instrument to try to reform what the mental health profession has so imperfectly created: As he tells us:

> There are right now, nearly three-quarters of a million patients in this nation's mental hospitals. Approximately 444,000 of them reside in state and county mental hospitals, the remainder in V.A. hospitals, and general hospitals with psychiatric wards. Many of them will be physically abused, a few will be raped or killed, but most of them will simply be ignored, left to fend for themselves in the cheerless corridors and barren back wards of the massive steel and concrete warehouses we—but not they—call hospitals. Each day thousands will die (the death rate by

age group is much higher in mental hospitals than outside) or be discharged, and other thousands will take their place.

During the coming year, one and a half million Americans will find themselves patients in a mental hospital, most against their wills. At the current admission rate, one out of every ten of us will someday be hospitalized for mental illness; admissions have doubled in the last fifteen years and are steadily rising. Already there are more patients in mental hospitals than in general hospitals, and three times as many patients as there are prisoners.

So vast an enterprise will occasionally harbor a sadistic psychiatrist or a brutal attendant, condemned even by his colleagues when discovered. But that is not the central problem. The problem, rather, is the enterprise itself.[3]

Is the community ready to give up such enterprises? There is one place on the North American continent where the death grip of institutionalism—this cycle of irrational ideology, misuse of resources, and ignorance of available technique—has been broken. In this case, there has been general community acceptance of the new system and it has worked well. This happened in southern Saskatchewan, where the hospital at Weyburn is no more. To our knowledge, this was the first time in North America that a plan was formulated and carried out to close a large mental hospital entirely in favor of a sectorized system of community services for the total population of the area once covered by the hospital. The principles underlying the development of this new system have been in operation for over ten years, successfully culminating in the closing of the hospital at Weyburn four years ago.

It closed in 1971, just 50 years after it had opened. Constructed to house a maximum of 1,000 patients, the seeds of its demise were built in, for even at its inception in 1921, the hospital contained an outpatient clinic. At the time, it was the only psychiatric resource for a population of 500,000 in a 54,000-square-mile area in the southern half of the province.

In 1930 a 20-bed psychiatric unit was constructed in the general hospital at Regina, the largest city in the service area. In spite of this, the population of the mental hospital grew until it finally reached the point where well over 2,500 patients were jammed within its confines under atrocious conditions. These matched and exceeded those described by Goffman,[8] Deutsch,[9] and Belknap[10] in similar institutions.

A turning point for the hospital was the appointment of the late D. G. McKerracher[11] as provincial director of mental health services by a newly elected socialist government under the leadership of T. C. Douglas. McKerracher was succeeded by the late F. S. Lawson[12] when the former became chairman and professor of psychiatry at the new Medical College of the University of Saskatchewan. These two men were the architects of the Saskatchewan Mental Health Services as we know them today.

The first specific relief to the mental hospital in Weyburn came when it was decided to transfer 1,000 mentally retarded patients to a new facility specifically designed for them. This brought the population of the hospital in Weyburn below the 2,000 mark.

The 1950s brought the tranquilizers and the humanization of the hospital by a new administration which placed considerable stress on the milieu. Outstanding contributions were made by Humphrey Osmond,[13] John and Elaine Cumming,[14,15] Ted Ayllon,[16] Robert Somer,[17,18] Hugo Ross, and Ted Weckowicz.[19] They transformed the hospital from one of the worst custodial institutions on the continent to one of the better mental hospitals (it was awarded the APA Silver Award in 1957 as a consequence). Simultaneously the number of inpatients declined and outpatient services expanded.

In 1956 a 24-bed psychiatric unit was established at the general

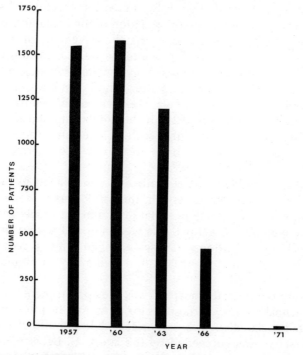

Figure 1. In-hospital census, December 31, 1957 to December 31, 1971.

hospital at Moose Jaw, the second largest city in the service area. In 1957, the "Saskatchewan Plan" was formulated by Lawson.[20] It called for the regionalization of the provincial psychiatric services into manageable service areas. Two new regional psychiatric services were established in Swift Current (1958) in the southwest corner of the province and Yorkton (1960) in the eastern part of the province.

In 1962–1963, a new administration was established under Fred Grunberg, Hugh Lafave, and Alec Stewart.[21,22,23] It was at this time that each of the five service areas defined under the Saskatchewan plan assumed total responsibility for psychiatric services in their areas, and this had a major impact on the hospital. Admissions and readmissions dropped dramatically (see Figures 1 and 2) and an increasing number of discharged patients were absorbed in the regional community programs (see Figure 3).

In 1965, with community services being developed and the hospital population down to 553, it became clear that the mental hospital could

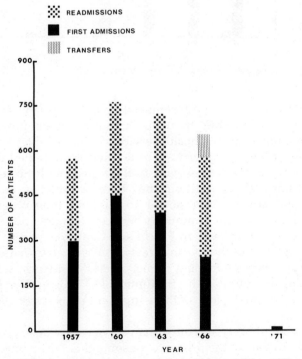

Figure 2. First admissions and readmissions, 1957 to 1971.

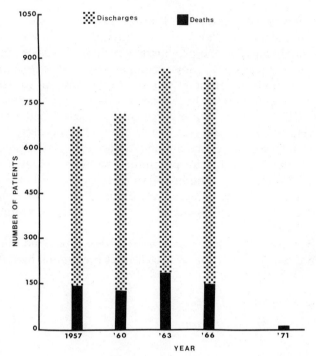

Figure 3. Deaths and discharges, 1957 to 1971.

be closed down. Plans were formulated accordingly, and in 1971 the hospital closed. This shift from an institution-based program to a regional community mental health service is seen in Tables I and II.

What must be emphasized about the figures in Table I is that the five programs provide total service to their areas with no recourse to any mental hospital. In addition, they have assimilated the so-called chronic mental patients from the old hospital into their programs.

Of the four inpatient community services, two are units in general hospitals. A third, the Yorkton Psychiatric Center, is part of a general hospital complex; and the fourth, Weyburn Psychiatric Center, moved in 1973 into a purpose-adapted former nurses' residence, which is to include an inpatient unit with a maximum of 63 beds in close proximity to the general hospital. None of these inpatient units resort to the use of locked doors.

Though community and outpatient services had been proliferating in the southern part of the province for some time, their impact on the seriously ill was negligible until the Saskatchewan plan was implemented in 1963. This seems akin to the general experience with community mental health centers and community programs in the United

Table I.  Number of Inpatients in General Hospitals and Community
Psychiatric Centers in All of Southern Saskatchewan[a]
(Pop. 500,000)

| Date | Weyburn | Moose Jaw General Hospital | Regina General Hospital, Munroe Wing | Yorkton Psychiatric Center | Swift Current Mental Health Center | Total |
|---|---|---|---|---|---|---|
| 9/31/62 | 1478 (Saskatchewan Hospital, Weyburn, closed 1971) | 20 | 25 | 8 | 0 | 1531 |
| 12/31/72 | 73 (Weyburn Psychiatric Center, opened 1963) | 15 | 28 | 24 | 0 | 140 |

[a]This includes Saskatchewan Hospital, Weyburn, before its closing.

States. Only infrequently or sporadically have they provided services to
people with serious disabilities. As a result, such people usually find
their way into mental hospitals. Admissions increase. Discharges
increase. Readmissions increase. And we have set in motion that awful
process: the revolving door.

Table II.  Outpatient Activities in Southern Saskatchewan Through 1971

| Year | Weyburn | Munroe | Moose Jaw | Yorkton | Swift Current | Total |
|---|---|---|---|---|---|---|
| Number of outpatients seen | | | | | | |
| 1962[a] | | | | | | 3,500+ |
| 1966 | 1,245 | 1,564 | 774 | 1,079 | 631 | 5,293 |
| 1970 | 1,193 | 1,792 | 702 | 1,257 | 670 | 5,614 |
| 1971 | 1,083 | 1,738 | 705 | 1,256 | 646 | 5,428 |
| Number of outpatient contacts | | | | | | |
| 1962[b] | | | | | | |
| 1966 | 10,815 | 12,925 | 7,312 | 12,487 | 4,182 | 47,721 |
| 1970 | 13,468 | 13,044 | 6,814 | 11,505 | 4,866 | 49,697 |
| 1971 | 13,540 | 17,103 | 9,262 | 12,612 | 5,257 | 57,774 |

[a]Total only.
[b]Figures not available.

Only when a team within a catchment area assumes total responsibility for all care within its boundaries do priorities shift so that true prevention and crisis-intervention programs are put into effect. When this shift occurs, it becomes possible to develop community services for the seriously ill. In Saskatchewan, these additional services ranged from group homes to sheltered workshops, from counseling services to rehabilitation programs. Their development contributed to a marked reduction in admissions and readmissions to the hospital.

Those in charge of putting the Saskatchewan plan into effect saw that reducing intake rather than pushing to discharge the existing patient population was the key to abolishing the big mental hospital. The three year drop of 73% in the inpatient population of Weyburn, from 1,519 in 1963 to 421 in 1966, resulted from a combination of many important factors,[24] but the decline in admissions and readmissions was the crucial one. It freed staff time to begin extensive rehabilitation programs which then prepared patients for return to their home communities. In turn their communities were better equipped to receive them as they expanded their services and gained experience. The plan was well under way by the end of 1964, and some opposition began to emerge from different quarters with different motivations.

*Patient's Relatives.* A number of patients' relatives, expecially in cases of long-hospitalized patients with families which had "closed ranks," began to become alarmed at the thought that the patient might "come home." This was particularly notable with geriatric patients. Much of this opposition occurred early in the program, and we learned from it that careful development of community programs must precede rapid rates of discharge. We also found that except in the case of married couples, it was usually preferable not to have former patients live with relatives. A series of living arrangements with different degrees of supervision was therefore developed as the alternative.

*Interested Citizens.* As the program expanded and as long-term patients were sent to the community, thus becoming more visible, humanitarian concern for their welfare began to be heard. Neighbors and citizen groups made complaints about instances where some patients had to live in substandard housing or did not have access to community programs and services. This mobilization of community support and advocacy for its disabled citizens can be the strength of a community program, and in Saskatchewan, it led to the development of better programs and improved standards.

*The Local Community.* The phasing out of the mental hospital was seen as a major threat to the economy of the small community where it was located. This was realistic, and we learned to coordinate our overall plans for patients' release with efforts to absorb retrained hospital staff into the new community programs, turn hospital facilities over to other health care and vocational training uses, and bring industrial jobs to the town.

*Professionals and Bureaucrats.* Some physicians, mostly those in general practice, became critical of the program and spoke of "wholesale discharge of chronic mental patients," claiming that this overtaxed the general health system. Others suspected the new community psychiatric program of overtaxing the social welfare system. These concerns were carefully evaluated and found not to be valid.[23]

Whether one looks at cost per client or at the overall provincial budget for psychiatric services, the community-based program is demonstrably less expensive. A 1967 study of the finances involving the cases of 458 chronic psychiatric patients discharged from Weyburn in 1964 and 1965 took into account the costs of welfare and other public assistance, psychiatric follow-up in the community, drugs, and rehospitalization; it was found that the total cost per client was $4.31 per day, in contrast to the $11.00 daily rate for hospital care.[25] Looking at southern Saskatchewan overall, the costs to the taxpayer for psychiatric services was $3,706,594 in 1962–1963; it was down about $0.5 million to $3,210,687 in 1972–1973, despite the rise in the cost of living during that ten-year period which witnessed the decline and eventual closing of the hospital.

When we learned to focus on prevention of admissions to mental hospitals, rather than on discharge, most opposition disappeared. Attempts to rush toward closing the mental hospital resulted in justifiable opposition, but there was no need to rush because a sensible pace would have brought the inevitable end of the hospital anyway. Had we taken five years instead of three to reduce the hospital population by three-quarters, most of the problems, minor as they were, could have been avoided. Thus there were mistakes made but implementation of the Saskatchewan plan was successful in the end as attested to by the following:

a. The readmission rate was low and remained so (Figure 2).
b. A succession of investigations which began as criticisms of the program ended by endorsing it.[22]
c. Information on outpatients provides an additional indicator of the program's activities and the amount of support it extended to patients and their families. In 1962, more than 3,500 outpatients were seen in the southern part of the province; by 1972 the number of people being followed had increased to 5,800.

The marked increase between 1966 and 1971, as shown by Table II, is evidence of the expansion of the community services program.

d. The outpatient figures do not adequately indicate the wealth of domiciliary services, home care programs, workshops, socialization centers, etc., that were developed. In addition, an advanced system of services for the elderly, which included home care services, group homes, low-rent apartments, senior citizens' villas, well-staffed nursing homes, extended-care facilities, and geriatric centers was elaborated by the departments of social services and health. These too had their impact on the delivery of psychiatric services, and in contrast to such services in the United States, were carefully maintained in Saskatchewan. Such services are required under provincial law to meet exacting standards, and do, for they are well supported by the public and by public funds.

e. Evidence from a number of independent research efforts showed that the program was successful.

One of the contributing factors to success was the visibility of the new program. Deficiencies were easily identified and exposed, and this led to swift corrective measures by the provincial authorities. Seldom was this the case when the provincial psychiatric program was based inside the institution, away from the eyes of the public. Patient neglect and dehumanization were easily hidden behind the walls of the mental hospital, and only when they reached grotesque proportions would scandal result in an investigation and the uncovering of the worst abuses. Rarely did this result in real change in the institutions and the furor would quickly die down. A great deal of interest in evaluating the program was shown by the hospital staff, by the federal and provincial governments, by citizen groups, and by the university. Thus, independent studies and observations—as well as studies by the staff—were essential parts of the outcome.* Studies are a necessary part of any such undertaking. Among other benefits, they provide data to help the press and the public understand what is happening.

In Saskatchewan, much thought went into how best to evaluate the approach to ensure that the plan was on the right track. It was felt that the most difficult area of the program concerned those hospitalized for a long time, since they had the dual problem of coping with their illness

---

*In other areas, such as New York and California, there has been a considerable push to deinstitutionalize, but here adequate research and evaluation of the outcome appear to be more the exception than the rule.

and of adjusting to community life after a period of institutionalization. It was, therefore, decided to study longitudinally all the long-term patients (those with continuous hospitalization of two years or more) who were discharged in 1963, 1964, and 1965. There were 508 such patients discharged from Weyburn during those years and they had spent an average of 18.2 years in the institution.

Two successive teams of investigators worked on the study,[26,27,28,29] each confirming each other's findings and refuting many of the concerns and criticisms which had been expressed by others. The researchers were funded by a federal grant and were not on the hospital payroll. The interviews were done by psychiatrists and social workers, each of whom spent one-and-one-half hours with each former patient and his or her closest relative. Many persons in the local community, including neighbors and those providing living arrangements, employers, were also interviewed about the program and the patient's adjustment.

The first team, under Dr. M. Herjanic, found that most of the discharged long-term patients were satisfied with the community arrangements and many voiced a strong desire never to return to the hospital. *Two-thirds* of those under 65 years of age had found jobs. In contrast to Wing's findings in Great Britain,[30] the people who had to deal directly with the former Weyburn patients in the community were generally pleased with them. As already noted, relatives were seldom asked to have patients with them. The result was that only one-third of the discharged patients studied lived with families. But wherever they lived, 80% of them were followed up regularly. Results showed there was a remarkable concurrence between the informants and investigators on how well patients were doing, and that much progress had been made by patients previously labeled "beyond recall."

The second team, under A. K. M. Fakhruddin,[28] showed that the positive results held up over the course of a five-year follow-up. Both research teams had been studying the long-term patient population, so an additional study of 115 consecutive discharges in 1965 was undertaken, in order to confirm that the other findings applied to all discharged patients regardless of length of hospitalization. Of the 100 patients who could be traced, 55 were employed and self-sufficient 1 year after discharge; another 16 were employed in sheltered settings; only 29 were not employed. Only 2 of the 115 had been readmitted to the hospital within a year of discharge.[31]

Nature seems to have designed the province of Saskatchewan as if it had in mind a comparative study. The province is neatly divided north and south by the Saskatchewan River as it flows from west to east. There are 500,000 people living in the north and 500,000 living in the south. There are two major cities, Regina in the south and Saskatoon in the north, and approximately 200,000 of the 500,000 people are concentrated in these cities. There was but one large public mental hospital in North Battleford in the north and the one at Weyburn in the south. The fact that the two populations were well matched on social, economic, and cultural factors adds to the symmetry and helps support the point that it was the decline in *admissions and readmissions*—rather than differences in the two populations—which dealt the death blow to the mental hospital.

As can be seen from Tables III, IV, and V, the hospital at North Battleford over a five-year period actually *discharged more people* than did the hospital at Weyburn. Yet the difference in the drop in their respective populations—much faster in the south—is striking. This would be even more the case were it not for the fact that during the fourth and fifth years, the drop in population at North Battleford accelerated as that area and that institution followed the example of the south and began to reduce admissions and readmissions. This served as further evidence of the success of the Weyburn program. Now, the size of the hospital population in the north has continued to decline to a point where North Battleford, for all intents and purposes, serves as the regional center for a portion of the northern part of the province, thus replicating much of what was accomplished at Weyburn.

At points along the way, there were often very real concerns on the part of families, staff, and the community about what the program at Weyburn was doing for patients. Although staff concerns were sometimes real, at other times they were masks for insecurity about their jobs. This anxiety was translated into fears on the part of the local community about the town's economic future, and this in turn led to apprehension on the part of politicians about the impact which continuation of the program might have on their chances for reelection.

Table III.   The Number of Inpatients at the Two Hospitals from 1961 to 1965

| Year | Hospital at North Battleford | Hospital at Weyburn |
|---|---|---|
| 1961 | 1,650 | 1,527 |
| 1962 | 1,613 | 1,478 |
| 1963 | 1,561 | 1,202 |
| 1964 | 1,401 | 796 |
| 1965 | 1,208 | 553 |

Table IV.   The Number of Discharges from the Two Hospitals from
1961 to 1965

| Year | Hospital at North Battleford | Hospital at Weyburn |
|---|---|---|
| 1961 | 849 | 762 |
| 1962 | 822 | 653 |
| 1963 | 830 | 679 |
| 1964 | 836 | 829 |
| 1965 | 733 | 582 |
| Total | 4070 | 3505 |

The chain of events resulted in several investigations which began with a bias against the program. For example, one investigation centered around a concern for the standard of homes in which former patients were living. Eventually, a delegation from the city of Weyburn met with the minister of health. As a result, "an ad hoc committee on the resettlement of mental patients was set up, consisting of four private citizens from Weyburn together with an associate professor of psychiatry, a general practitioner, a representative of the Provincial Department of Social Welfare and one from the Canadian Mental Health Association."[22]

Though they began as critics, at the conclusion of their investigation, they were "impressed by the exciting possibilities of caring for the mentally ill with minimal custodial care, and by the considerable degree of community tolerance shown towards these discharged patients. The apparent appreciation of the majority of patients at being out of the hospital was similarly striking, as was the reiteration on the part of landladies, that many of these patients had improved to a large degree as a result of their new environment." On the other hand, the

Table V.   Total Admissions to the Two Hospitals from 1961 to 1965
(Includes Readmissions)

| Year | Hospital at North Battleford | Hospital at Weyburn |
|---|---|---|
| 1961 | 878 | 852 |
| 1962 | 990 | 833 |
| 1963 | 1006 | 717 |
| 1964 | 868 | 519 |
| 1965 | 749 | 468 |
| Total | 4491 | 3389 |

investigators were "distressed by the variety of standards of care for these patients." As a result, the committee recommended clearly defined standards for group homes and the establishment of training programs for group home operators; these reforms were put into effect in the latter part of 1966.

The committee went far beyond this, as its following recommendations indicate:

1. We recommend that the Saskatchewan Plan, based on a complete regionalization of psychiatric care in order to make psychiatric attention available locally, be fully and enthusiastically endorsed by the Government of Saskatchewan, and that the government proceed immediately to establish the necessary facilities and staff for the implementation of the program on a province-wide basis.

2. We recommend that those responsible for the care of mentally ill in the province of Saskatchewan be commended and encouraged. In particular, the staff of the Saskatchewan Hospital, Weyburn have tacked a very difficult problem with imagination, courage and initiative. On the whole, when the magnitude of the problem is considered, it is remarkable how smoothly the program has worked despite obvious problems of adjustment amongst staff, patients, relatives, and the community at large.

Subsequent investigations would also begin as criticism of a facet of the program but would end by assisting in the correction of the problem under study and by endorsing the total plan.

The feasibility and desirability of abandoning mental hospitals as a modality of services in a public psychiatric program is still debated in other jurisdictions in Canada, the United States, and the United Kingdom.[32,33,34,35,36] However, the province of Saskatchewan has completely done away with its traditional mental hospital in the southern part of the province and the new ideology of community services has extended to the rest of the province.

In summary, what distinguishes the Saskatchewan program and in large part accounts for its success is that the drop in the hospital population did not result from any administrative fiat restricting admissions to it. Nor did it result from large numbers of unprepared patients being dumped on communities ill equipped to receive them. Rather, as a result of declining admissions through the provision of alternative community services, the inpatient populations dropped. Extensive rehabilitation programs (these included the use of behavior modification techniques and "work for pay" programs) were then developed to prepare long-term patients[37] for discharge. Careful planning assisted their assimilation into their home communities by the team servicing that area. This assured extensive follow-up and the development of specialized programs to meet their needs.

## *Ideology*

Can the experience in the microcosm of Saskatchewan be repeated elsewhere? It is clear to us that it can. The fact that it has not happened in other places relates less to the question of community readiness than to a question of what social structures maintain the institution in this society.

It is the ideology of banishment—of dispatching disabled citizens to total institutions on the pretext that they are able to offer care when in fact their purpose is to keep them out of sight and out of mind. This practice is justified through the myth that the present state of knowledge limits our ability to do more for the mentally "disturbed."

Communities have been allowed and encouraged to export their most pressing human service problems, along with some of their resources and local control. On the one hand, in small communities this is done with accompanying rhetoric about the need for expertise, specialization, and facilities beyond the capabilities of the community itself; at the same time the cities—rich in these capacities—are shipping their troubled individuals off to "a place in the country." An ideology that allows this to go on is false and irrational.

Society holds firmly to the practice of institutionalization, despite change in many other areas of values and behavior; a high regard for "progress" helped this society overcome major obstacles in mobilizing the resolve, the technology, and the money needed to undertake projects of questionable value such as building a continent-wide network of high-speed highways and a spectacular space exploration program within a few decades. Yet the same society has made no similar commitment on a problem of immediate concern to every community: namely, to put an end to the practice of exiling some of its members in the name of treatment.

Support must be rallied around the principle that each community take care of its own people, using its own human and financial resources as far as possible, and that when the community is not able to undertake this complete responsibility, efforts and resources should be coordinated in specific and limited ways with neighboring areas. This is not to deny the importance of national and international exchange of ideas, experience, and research results, nor of state and federal funds to enable local communities to implement their plans and programs. But a viable system of human services must begin with local responsibility and must renounce the expedient of exporting its problem people.

Frequently there is a lag between the time when a society achieves a technological advance, and when an awareness of its nontechnological potential develops. In the realm of human services, a basic technology for assisting seriously disabled individuals in vastly more humane ways and at similar or lesser cost has existed for over two decades. Community services have been demonstrated which obviate the need to remove individuals from their home communities to mental hospitals. What is still frequently lacking is the emergence of a social consciousness which will activate the commitment to implementation on a broad front.

Why should this lag in human services last for such a long time? Why do communities continue to exile thousands from their midst into distant, overcrowded, scandal-ridden institutions?

A community's readiness to take a fresh approach in carrying out its responsibilities depends to a great extent on the values held by the society of which it is a part. We would not deny that a locality has a role in shaping the values of its larger society; however, the contribution which any single community can make is limited, since the prevailing value is usually more than a simple summing up of the contributed parts.

Thus, though a community can sometimes accomplish a great deal on its own, if its aspirations go against the grain of the overall society, that community will have a much harder time accomplishing its goals.

The real revolution in care for the mentally ill cannot stem only from the discovery of more effective medication or the ultimate causes of schizophrenia or more advanced architectural design. The basic change must be rooted in the recognition that society has supported an undeniable policy of banishment and that this policy and the ideology behind it must be abandoned in favor of new programs of support services in the community for all who need assistance and an acceptance of local responsibility.

When we are asked, "Is the community ready?" our response is to ask the professionals, the politicians, and the bureaucrats if they are willing to take on leadership roles to ensure that there is acceptance and understanding, at the societal level, of the worth of good community-based mental health services. Instead, as a result of ignorance, malice, self-interest, or expedience, they have too often reinforced the old practices and undercut the new by fostering the belief that it is the community that is holding up the parade.

## Techniques

The question of readiness must be posed primarily to the professionals, politicians, and bureaucrats. Among these we would zero in on the professionals, who more often than not have been the ones to ask the public to accept half-baked ideas such as revolving door policies as substitutes for the institution. They have been primarily responsible for allowing large numbers of unprepared patients to be dumped from institutions. Often this has been into areas adjacent to them. These quickly become oversaturated with seriously disabled people who have few if any ties to the community in which they find themselves.

Where instead a society has accepted the value of preventing the exile of its citizens to institutions, and where resources are available and adequate to the task,* the professional in the field becomes the focal point for success or failure at the community level.

Unfortunately, failure has been more common than success. And where the professional is responsible, failures fall into two general categories. In the first, some professionals do not accept the ideology, frequently rejecting it in favor of maintaining their own self-interests. In the second, they accept the ideology but lack the know-how to develop community-based services.

In the first category and despite all empirical evidence to the contrary, there are mental health professionals who continue to look the other way. Atkinson[38] is not convinced by the evidence that "hospitalization is categorically stigmatizing." Yet Rabkin, reviewing the research done on attitudes toward mental illness concludes, "By 1969, it was clearly established that mental illness is feared and those labelled as mental patients were disliked and avoided by most people."[39] The public was more willing than mental health professionals to define a broad range of behavior as normal. But hospitalization becomes a key factor in changing attitudes and labeling a person as "mentally ill."

The public response is then "characteristically negative and rejecting." The label usually leads to diminished standing in the eyes of the community; a circumstance that, of course, exacerbated whatever problems were initially present. The effects of the label are often severe. "Being an ex-mental patient is more of a liability than being an ex-criminal in pursuit of housing, jobs, friends." Studies in the early 1970s showed that despite minor gain, this attitude still prevailed and that the general public was still apprehensive about ex-mental patients. Nonetheless, they believed that the labeling could be avoided. There was nearly unanimous agreement that "a lot can be done to prevent mental illness." The majority believed that mental patients are better off in the community than in a mental hospital.

In the face of this, Atkinson can still dismiss as overstatement the

---

*As will be discussed in the section on resources, it takes no more to run good community programs than it takes to run the institution it can replace.

works of Goffman, Sarbin, Mendel, Ennis, and others on the stigmatization of ex-mental patients and can reject the ideology.

In this same category, many psychiatrists working in community programs, whether based in mental health centers or psychiatric units of general hospitals, have been unprepared to give up the convenience of exporting their treatment failures or their problem patients to the mental hospital. Rather than struggle with the new challenge of taking service into the community itself, they have found it easier to egg the community on—giving special attention to the media and the politicians with claims that the total institution is still needed for the protection of the community since alternatives are not available. They have often maintained that the public has a sterotype of mental illness as being characterized by "violence and assaultive behavior"[40] and have played into these ideas and used them to resist the development of community services.

These same professionals drag their feet when it comes to developing new plans and programs in their communities. In this way, they ensure that what they say about the need for the institution in fact becomes the case.

Such professionals who make a case for retention of mental hospitals and object to the release of patients from them are often motivated by the prospect of losing a convenience. As it stands, they are able to banish their most difficult clients by virtue of their control of admissions and of open-ended retention of patients in institutions. Community psychiatrists of this stripe want to have their cake and eat it too.

Top administrators in the mental hospitals constitute another group of professionals who are opposed to the community mental health ideology. They are supported by elements in the central state bureaucracy who have strong incentives for maintaining the institution since they provide them with status, power, and material comfort.

Further support comes from other professionals in the institution at all levels. They goad employees, unions, and townspeople who fear that any change in the status quo of the mental hospital will cause loss of jobs locally. This institutionalization of the staff—no less than that of the patients—is accompanied by a fear of being rapidly returned to the "community." The professional—in the face of the need for change—should play a key role in planning and implementing the transition in a way that minimizes its impact on the employee and the local community. Instead, professionals in this situation often take an opposite approach.

In the second category are those who are supportive of community-based services in principle, but who fail because they lack knowledge of the techniques available, lack ability to apply them or to adapt them to a particular situation.

Kris,[41] Herz,[42] Pasamanick,[43] Langsley,[44] Marx,[45] Mendel,[46] and the Saskatchewan experience[21,22] have clearly demonstrated techniques available to us which are superior to the mental hospital. These techniques must be understood by the professionals applying them at the community level. It is grossly unfair to ask a community to be a part of a new system unless services are well planned and well executed to suit its particular needs.

As was noted in our review of the Saskatchewan experience, programs must cover a wide range from workshops to socialization clubs, from living arrangements to health care centers. Professionals, adept as administrators, capable of spanning this range of programming and able to relate to all elements in a community, are vital to success. Beyond this, an additional quality often demanded of professionals and programs is an ability to adapt to rapidly changing times and trying circumstances.

It may be useful to examine in some detail an example of one such adaptive approach. It deals with the problem of coordination of community-based services that rely heavily on the collaborative model. "Modular programming,"[47] as the technique is called, consists of flexible structuring of environments through varied arrangements of time, space, and people to meet the full range of the personal needs of a disabled individual, his family, and the community. Within its framework, such clients and their families are helped to plan their lives and activities in terms of day, evening, and overnight modules. These component sections of the 24-hour day are designed to reflect the ebb and flow of daily living, providing a way of working with individuals and of planning programs for them so that all the tasks do not fall on one individual, family, group, or agency. Modular programming reorients care and treatment away from total institutionalization and such older concepts as residential or nonresidential, inpatient or outpatient.

The daytime module is given first consideration and focuses on educational, prevocational, and vocational activities, depending on one's age. The evening and weekend modules concentrate on opportunities for socialization, recreation, and the development of self-help skills. The overnight module becomes the base from which the other activities are pursued: a place to sleep, to relax, to unwind—a place to call home.

The ease with which the overnight module can be provided depends largely on the success of fully developing the other two modules. If adequate day and evening modules are available, the service expectation of the overnight module is clearly defined and limited. When the tasks are distributed among different service providers under different auspices, the patient can benefit from variety; and providers benefit by offering that service for which they are best equipped.

A basic tenet of this programming is that successive modules should occur in different locations except in the case of very young or acutely ill persons. This establishes a rhythm to life in which people move from one setting to another—from their home to their place of work or study, and thence to their place of recreation, and back again.

This concept in a sense is the antithesis of how programming is structured in the total institution. It aims at a sharing between the program and the family instead of the old "all or nothing" model in which a family had all the responsibility for its members or else it dumped a member in the mental hospital and then had no responsibility.

New approaches such as modular programming must be adapted and elaborated in ways which meet the needs of communities and their members. It is not enough that professionals subscribe to the idea of community services. They must be creative in developing new techniques to censure their success.

This must be taken to the point that professionals who cling to outmoded ideas about the efficacy of mental hospitals are discredited by being confronted with community programs which speak for themselves.

## Community (or Lack Thereof)

What do we mean by "community"? This is a basic question, because a "sense of community"—a sense of common interest or shared identity—among people is certainly prerequisite to the existence of any notion that they should not exile those among them who need help. There are many definitions of community—some of them popular, some academic, some official, and many overlapping. Regester notes some implications for community mental health programs of the particular meanings which are given to the word *community*.[48]

In regard to the planning and delivery of human services, we must first think pragmatically of community in geographical terms: Where and for what population are services needed?

But it is necessary to go further. Although people usually talk of a city, a town, or a village as being a community, the key points in defining a "sense of community" go beyond political boundaries, population, size, and location.

Stories are frequently told of city dwellers who live near but not in touch with each other, of people in trouble being ignored by dozens who have heard their cries for help; of next-door neighbors never becoming acquainted. Thus, while "community" implies physical proximity—people living near enough to each other to keep in contact—it must also be defined in social terms: a shared set of values and an established pattern of interaction among people; a sharing of common interests and a willingness to share in the tasks done in pursuit of these interests; and a concern for the welfare of all those joined together in these interests and tasks. It is obvious that few if any places in the world qualify on all counts of this social definition of community. But some localities large and small come close enough so that the development of community-based services as we have described them can go on.

An ideology of local responsibility is essential and an adequate sense of community is a necessary precursor to this. Places without it will not be fertile fields in which a positive ideology can take root and community-based programs will not have a good chance of success. In some cases, the state of disorganization of a town or neighborhood may be so severe as to preclude any effective action by large enough numbers of residents, by their political representatives, or by outside mental health professionals. These are places where people are struggling to maintain a marginal existence with regard to the basics of food, clothing, and shelter in the absence of a workable set of norms and with little or no commitment to being mutually supportive. In our opinion, some mental health professionals have been overoptimistic about what they have to contribute to the process of change in settings where there is a state of near anomie.

In a megalopolis where this is sometimes the situation, disproportionate numbers of casualties are produced and it is here that much of the criticism has been generated against the community model.[49] Cries of failure might as well be directed against any of the services in such settings, whether we are talking about law enforcement, mass transit systems, health care, or education. Here the very fabric of the society has come unraveled. A realistic look then at the problem may lead to the conclusion that mental health services must be moved down the list of priorities; community organization must be put to work first on the survival needs of the area, as far as the people and their representatives are concerned.

In the meantime, successful programs in other jurisdictions cannot but have an enhancing effect on the communities where so much more needs to be done. The fact that in some localities such programs cannot be successful at this juncture is not a valid excuse to delay the growth of community services in all areas. It is our view that in most North American communities, a sufficient sense of "community" exists or can be rallied to support noninstitutional mental health services, and that the community *is* ready.

## Resources

If ideology determines the outline of human services, then resources *must* certainly be the oils which are necessary to bring the painting to life. Without resources, we have but the idea and the ideal. (Unfortunately, the analogy of services as artistry has all too often given way to a less attractive comparison, with ideology the battleground and resources the prize being sought.)

At a time when total institutions were seen as having a valid function, resources flowed to them, though never in proportion to their increase in population as more and more people were banished to their care. The concept of economy of scale led institutions to grow to unmanageable size till even the most strenuous efforts at containment became futile. This lunacy was epitomized by a 10,000-bed "bedlam" on Long Island.

Attempts to shore up the institutions as scale led to scandal took the form of more building and pleas for more staff. When it was suggested that alternatives be developed, the common approach was to divert a fraction (and almost always a ridiculously small fraction) of available resources from the institution into inadequate programs charged to function as "community services."

This approach had the seeds of failure sown into it on two counts. First, the community was seldom able to generate adequate services in its midst because adequate funding was not provided. And as with any other investment, money must precede service.

The other fallacy in these token community programs was that because they were so severly limited in scope and function, they could only operate in the shadow of a large, established institution which was more than ready to take on the task of "backup" or "court of last resort." The disproportionate flow of money to the institution makes this an easy role to fulfill.

The combination of meager resources to apply in the community plus the continuation of a readily available place for banishment results in a community service program which is neither motivated nor financially positioned to generate a range of services adequate to the task of preventing admissions and readmissions to the mental hospital. The excuse that more resources are necessary within the mental health system to bring about the total shift to community services is just that— an excuse. The change from one system to another can generally be accomplished within the limits of existing mental health allocations— seldom is new money needed.

Over the past twenty years, we have been confronted with examples—affirmed and reaffirmed—of the outcome of add-on "community teams" or community treatment center that also represent add-on costs to the taxpayer. The usual experience is that initially some services are performed for a few people. In a short period of time, one of two directions is taken. The first is that unmet needs will mount in proportion to the shortcomings of the program, and the old cliché will once again be demonstrated that "community services can only do so much—the institution is still needed." This "confirmation" then provides justification for maintaining funding in community services at low or even reduced levels, and institutional dependency continues with renewed vigor—perhaps having made a successful argument for new buildings and additional staffing as a consequence.

The second possibility is that the attempt to intercept and assist people with serious problems is not even initiated. (Sadly, in the few instances where community programs have been reasonably funded, they have often adopted this stance.) In this model, no one ever expects or claims that the community program is to be more than a "hand-holding" center. People with serious disabilities bypass the center altogether and seek admission to institutional care, or at most the community program serves as a sorting device.

Unfortunately, the ultimate effect of this is the same. The necessity for continuation of the institutions is "affirmed," as is the limitation of community services, and this is subsequently reflected in the allocation of resources.

The popular term *outreach* makes the point: Activities are concentrated in the institution and an extension to the community is established as a channel of communication rather than as the principle means for actually performing the tasks.

At some point, a commitment must be made on the part of the society that community services will be provided for the mentally ill, including the most severely disabled. Until such a commitment is made, the community has an obligation to be unready; until the major share of resources for services to the mentally ill is set to the task of developing programs which preclude the necessity of sending people to mental hospitals, the community cannot be ready.

A thousand excuses can be found not to do this, most commonly that resources cannot be stretched to maintain facilities as well as to initiate meaningful community services. This argument against dein-stitutionalization cannot be accepted. Reducing funds to the institution can hasten its end. Simultaneously, the funds must be reallocated to communities and community service programs, ready and willing to take up the task. Only in this way can the cycle of support for the old ideology be broken.

## Conclusion

Since services in the community can be adequately rendered at reasonable cost without making unreasonable demands on the individual served, his family, the community, and the society at large, why should the community not be ready?

There is certainly a need to accumulate much more experience with community-based services which meet the needs of all the mentally disabled in a given population. But the evidence to date supports community-based services as superior to mental hospital programs or equal to them at reduced cost. There is no evidence to show that the mental hospital is superior to community-based services.

At a time when the technology was less developed than it is today, successful programs were implemented in Saskatchewan. There, a public mental hospital system was phased out in favor of a community-based system of services to a total population. The fact that this could work where it did, when it did, is testimony to the feasibility of what is advocated.

Why is there still so much confusion, resistance, and opposition to the idea of closing mental hospitals? Part of the explanation lies in the complexity of a pluralistic society, where it becomes inordinately difficult to get all of the necessary elements harnessed together and to keep them working in tandem for long enough to accomplish the task.

For example, when the professionals of the Joint Commission on Mental Health launched the movement for community-based services, there seemed to be a supporting ideology and good acceptance on the part of politicians and the bureaucracy. Much of the resistance came from elsewhere within the professional mental health ranks. By the time enough of these professionals had come into line, a backlash was beginning to develop in some communities and support in the political sector was starting to weaken, largely as a result of half-hearted implementation of poorly planned programs and the overselling of new programs.

And so it is that at least one critical element has always managed to stay out of step, halting or slowing the development of a good system of noninstitutional services. Those who would burden the community with full responsibility for the painfully slow pace of change in services are searching for a scapegoat. If all other elements would do their part, communities would not represent an obstacle to the implementation of programs that would spell the demise of the mental hospital—a demise that is long overdue.

The communities are ready. Many of them are waiting. Some of them are pushing. They cannot be used as excuses for not moving ahead. Let us look to our politicians and our bureaucrats and most of all to our mental health professionals. They have been vested with a full measure of authority—we hope for a matching level of responsibility.

## References

1. Bigelow, N., & Roberts, E. The state hospital golf course. *Psychiatric Quarterly Supplement,* 1968, **42**(2), 321–336.
2. Wasted money—Wasted lives: A report on the New York State Department of Mental Hygiene. *Albany* (New York) *Times Union,* May 4--10, 1975.
3. Ennis, B. *Prisoners of psychiatry.* New York: Harcourt Brace Jovanovich, 1972.
4. Solomon, H. Presidential address, American Psychiatric Association, 1958.
5. *Action for mental health.* Report by Joint Commission on Mental Illness and Health, Washington, D.C., 1961.
6. *More for the mind.* Report of the Committee on Psychiatric Services, Toronto, Ontario, 1963.
7. Annual report. Royal Commission on Health Services, Ottawa, 1964.
8. Goffman, E. *Asylums.* New York: Doubleday, 1961.
9. Deutsch, A. *The shame of the states.* New York: Harcourt Brace, 1948.
10. Belknap, I. *Human problems of a state mental hospital.* New York: McGraw-Hill, 1956.
11. McKerracher, D. G., Smith, C. M., & Coburn, F. E. General practice psychiatry: An account of two Canadian experiments. *Lancet,* Nov. 13, 1965, 1005–1007.
12. Lawson, F. S. From institution to community: The Saskatchewan Plan. *Canadian Nurse,* 1967, **68**, 26–29.
13. Osmond, H., & Smythies, J. Schizophrenia: A new approach. *Journal of Mental Science,* 1952, **98**, 309–315.
14. Cumming, J., & Cumming, E. *Closed ranks.* Cambridge: Howard University Press, 1957.
15. Cummings, J., & Cumming, E. *Ego and milieu.* New York: Atherton Press, 1962.
16. Ayllon, T., & Michael, J. The psychiatric nurse as behavioral engineer. *Journal of the Experimental Analysis of Behavior,* 1959, **2**, 323–334.

17. Somer, R. The mental hospital in the small community. *Mental Hygiene,* 1958, **42,** 488–496.
18. Somer, R., & Ross, H. Social interaction on a geriatric ward. *International Journal of Social Psychiatry,* 1958, **4,** 128–133.
19. Weckowicz, T., Somer, R., & Hall, R. Distance constancy in schizophrenic patients. *Journal of Mental Science,* 1958, **104,** 1174–1182.
20. Lawson, F. S. The Saskatchewan plan. *Mental Hospitals,* 1957, **5,** 27–31.
21. Lafave, H. G., Stewart, A., & Grunberg, F. Community care of the mentally ill: Implementation of the Saskatchewan plan. *Community Mental Health Journal,* 1968, **4,** 37–45.
22. Stewart, A., Lafave, H. G., Grunberg, F., & Herjanic, M. Problems in phasing out a large public psychiatric hospital. *American Journal of Psychiatry,* 1968, **125,** 120–126.
23. Cassel, W. A., Grunberg, F., & Frazier, H. N. The discharged chronic patient: Utilization of health resources—a preliminary report. *Canadian Psychiatric Association Journal,* **13**(23), 1968.
24. Lafave, H. G., Herjanic, M., & Grunberg, F. One-year follow-up of 67 chronic psychiatric patients. *Canadian Psychiatric Association Journal,* 1966, **2**(3), 205.
25. Cassell, W. A., Smith, C. M., Grunberg, F., Boan, J. A., & Thomas, R. Comparing costs of hospital and community care. *Hospital and Community Psychiatry,* 1972, **23,** 197–200.
26. Herjanic, J., Stewart, A., & Hales, R. C. The chronic patient in the community—A two year follow up of 339 chronic patients. *Canadian Psychiatric Association Journal,* 1968, **13,** 231–235.
27. Herjanic, M., Hales, R. C., & Stewart, A. Does it pay to discharge the chronic patient? A two year follow up of 338 chronic patients. *Acta Psychiatrica Scandinavica,* 1969, **45,** 53–61.
28. Fakhruddin, A. K. M., Manjooran, A., Nair, N. P. V., & Neufeldt, A. A five year outcome of discharged chronic psychiatric patients. *Canadian Psychiatric Association Journal,* 1972, **17,** 433–435.
29. Lafave, H. G., Herjanic, M., & Grunberg, F. One year follow up of 67 chronic psychiatric patients. *Canadian Psychiatric Association Journal,* 1966, **11,** 205–212.
30. Wing, J. K., & Hailey, A. M. (Eds.). *Evaluating a community psychiatry service.* London: Oxford University Press, 1972.
31. Luterbach, E., Luterbach, R., Lafave, H. G., & Stewart, A. *The job status of 115 discharged psychiatric patients.* Unpublished paper, 1968.
32. Mendel, W. M. *Dismantling the mental hospital.* Academic debate, Canadian Psychiatric Association meeting, Vancouver, June 1973.
33. Community psychiatry: When the rhetoric had to stop (Editorial). *Lancet,* July 21, 1973.
34. Gottesfeld, H. (Ed.). *The critical issues in community mental health.* New York: Behavioral Publications, 1972.
35. Vail, D. J. *Dehumanization and the institutional career.* Springfield, Illinois: Charles C Thomas, 1966.
36. Weiner, S., Bird, B. J., & Arthur Bolton Associates. *Process and impacts of the closing of DeWitt State Hospital.* Menlo Park, California: Stanford Research Institute, 1973.
37. Stewart, A., Lafave, H. G., & Grunberg, F. *Halving the population of a large public psychiatric hospital in two years.* Paper read at 122nd annual meetings of the American Psychiatric Association, Atlantic City, New Jersey, May, 1966.
38. Atkinson, R. M. Current and emerging models of residential psychiatric treatment, with special reference to the California situation. *American Journal of Psychiatry,* 1975, **132**(4), 391–396.

39. Rabkin, J. Public attitudes toward mental illness: A review of the literature. *Schizophrenia Bulletin,* 1974, **10,** 9–33.
40. Spiro, H. R., Siassi, I., Crocetti, G. The issue of contact with the mentally ill. *American Journal of Public Health,* 1974, **64,** 887–879.
41. Kris, E. Prevention of rehospitalization through relapse control in a day hospital. In M. Greenblatt, D. J. Levinson, & G. L. Klerman (Eds.), *The mental patient in transition.* Springfield, Illinois: Charles C Thomas, 1961, pp. 155–162.
42. Herz, M. I., Endicott, J., Spitzer, R. L., et al. Day versus inpatient hospitalization: A controlled study. *American Journal of Psychiatry,* 1971, **127,** 1371–1382.
43. Pasamanick, B., Scarpitti, F. R., & Dinitz, S. *Schizophrenics in the community.* New York: Appleton-Century-Crofts, 1967.
44. Langsley, D. G., & Kaplan, D. M. *The treatment of families in crisis.* New York: Grune and Stratton, 1968.
45. Marx, A. J., Test, M. A., & Stein, L. I. Extrahospital management of severe mental illness: Feasibility and the effects of social functioning. *Archives of General Psychiatry,* 1973, **29,** 505–511.
46. Mendel, W. M. Effect of length of hospitalization on rate and quality of remission from acute psychotic episodes. *Journal of Nervous and Mental Disease,* 1966, **143,** 226–233.
47. Woodhouse, R., & Lafave, H. G. *Modular programming: Basis for collaboration.* Schenectady, New York, 1974. (Mimeo)
48. Regester, D. C. Community mental health—for whose community? *American Journal of Public Health,* 1974, **64,** 886–893.
49. Kolb, L. C. Where the work is done. *Psychiatric Annals,* May 1974, **4** (5), 8–13.

# 13

# Whither the State Hospital?

## Issues and Trends in Mental Health Services Delivery

PAUL I. AHMED

The cost-benefit issues in mental health are becoming increasingly important. Now that making health services available to all citizens through health insurance has become a domestic priority, inclusion of mental health services in the coverage is almost a certainty. This will create both new demands for mental health services as well as demands for evaluation of the benefits provided.

Not too far in the future, then, not only consumers but taxpayers will be asking many questions about benefits received from mental health services. At that time I fear the profession will not be terribly convincing in giving its usual explanations that mental health services are really different from other health services and, therefore, should not be examined under a cost–benefit microscope.

Furthermore, those in the field of mental health may have to face up to the fact that they cannot meet the call for psychological and social help for all of the sick, the poor, the underachieving, the frustrated, the underemployed or the unemployed, and the claustrophobic residents of our cities.

In today's changing world, as we are moving from a "consumption-oriented" society to a more "utilitarian" way of life due to energy and raw material shortages, the fabric of our society is under a great

PAUL I. AHMED • Professor, Southeastern University, Washington, D.C. 20024 strain. It may eventually lead to changes in the value system of our citizens as well as a move from a production-oriented society priding itself on the planned obsolescence of what it produces to a more "service-oriented" economy. These changes are enormous. They can bring adjustment problems to all—the strong and the more vulnerable as well. And so we may need more research and training funds to train mental health professionals, but more important, mental health professionals may have to set up priorities and make judgments about what is possible to deal with and what is not possible.

Against the backdrop of these national changes, goals of specific mental health service delivery remain unfulfilled. President Kennedy's promise years ago that we would have community mental health care for all is not yet a reality. Out of 2,000 community mental health centers needed, only 450 or so are operating at present. The new extension of the Community Mental Health Centers Act would bring some new resources, but we cannot expect a federally financed effort for networks of community care all across the nation in the near future. States and localities must now take up the mission of establishing more community mental health centers.

Another change in the mental health service picture has been the steady decline since the mid-1950s in the number of resident patients in state mental hospitals, as shown in Table I.

These statistics highlight two facts: the staff patient ratio has changed from 1:3 to 1:1, and there is a continuing discrepancy between per diem costs in general hospitals and mental hospitals.

A liquidation of state hospitals has taken place at an increasing rate in the states of California, Massachusetts, Ohio, Washington, and elsewhere. At the same time, state hospital property has risen in value, and in many localities former hospitals are now being used for community colleges, nursing homes, etc. On the other hand, the sad fact is emerging that mental hospitals are viewed as a major, if not the only, new resource of funds to develop additional community mental health programs.

Table I.  Patient–Staff Ratios and Patient Care Costs[a]

|                          | 1959     | 1972     |
| ------------------------ | -------- | -------- |
| Patient population       | 542,721  | 275,995  |
| Staff population         | 174,218  | 219,777  |
| Patient-care cost per diem | $4.44  | $20.68   |

[a]Joint Commission on Mental Health and Illness, 1959, 1972.

A new concept in mental hospitals has developed in the last decade. As the CCMHCs have taken over responsibility for aftercare and rehabilitation, hospitals have assumed new roles in community outreach and treatment programs. Thus, hospitals have come to adopt more of a CCMHC character. The state hospitals have also learned the intricacies of financing, and now they collect fees from Medicare, Medicaid, and welfare patients. The resource development and collection capacity of mental hospitals have substantially increased through third-party payments, contract and grant money, etc. Recently, there have also been major changes in the profile of patients receiving care in mental hospitals. In 1971, for example, one-half of all patient-care episodes for patients 65 years old and over in psychiatric facilities took place in state hospitals. Between 1962 and 1972, alcohol disorders and other substance abuse disorders have increased substantially in hospital admissions, as shown in Table II.

The substantial increases for the rates per 100,000 population during a 10-year period for those under 15 and for the 15–24 age group, and decreases in the 55–64 and 65–over groups point to our dilemma. The young people under 15 and those of college age (15–24) are getting more and more treatment in mental hospitals, while those with the least employment potential, i.e., the 55–64 and 65–over groups, are receiving it in the community. The reason is perhaps obvious. With substantial increases in alcoholism and drug abuse rates, the community is just not able to provide detoxification facilities to all who need them, and some must be referred to state mental hospitals. The comparison of diagnostic distribution of first admissions to state and community mental hospitals during the past decade reveals alcohol disorders as the leading diagnostic category in 1972 for all age groups, and schizophrenia and brain syndrome dropping in percentages. The figures for first admissions for all age groups are shown in Table III for the years 1972 and 1973.

Table II.   Percent Distribution of Admissions with No Prior
Inpatient and Psychiatric Care to State and County Mental Hospitals
for Selected Diagnostic Groups[a]

|                            | 1962 | 1965 | 1969 | 1972 |
|----------------------------|------|------|------|------|
| Alcohol disorders[b]       | 15.0 | 16.9 | 25.7 | 26.1 |
| Drug abuse disorders[b]    | 1.3  | 2.5  | 3.9  | 6.5  |
| Neuroses                   | 9.4  | 11.0 | 12.1 | 12.4 |
| Personality disorders      | 9.1  | 10.6 | 8.9  | 10.5 |

[a]Biometry Branch, NIMH.
[b]Includes those in corresponding brain syndrome category.

Table III.   Percent Distribution of All
Admissions for All Age Groups in a State and
Mental Hospital for Selected Diagnostic Groups[a]

|                        | 1972 | 1973 |
|------------------------|------|------|
|                        | %    | %    |
| Alcohol disorders      | 23.2 | 23.7 |
| Schizophrenia          | 30.7 | 30.8 |
| Depression             | 10.1 | 9.8  |
| Organic brain syndrome | 7.8  | 7.3  |
| Drug disorders         | 5.4  | 5.3  |

[a]Admissions and resident patients at the end of the year in
state and county mental hospitals: 1972, 1973. Biometry
Branch, NIMH.

Forty percent of the resident hospital population (the ratio has
remained constant since 1955) are schizophrenic and probably have
been in hospitals for a long time.

Thirty percent of the releases from state mental hospitals in 1969
were referred to nursing homes or homes for the aged. If additional
community facilities, such as halfway houses, nursing homes, etc.,
were available, more patients could be released to the community.

Accelerated decline in the resident rate in mental hospital population does not really signify the lack of need for sheltered care facilities.
As a matter of fact, we may have had no decline in the populations
needing sheltered care, but only a decline in resident rates in state
hospitals. In 1964, there were 249,000 patients with mental disorders in
nursing homes. In 1972, the number was 640,000. Thus, we still had
almost 900,000 patients in 1972 with psychiatric disorders in sheltered-
care facilities. Given the recent decline in the number of nursing homes
available due to certification problems under Medicare, the resident
populations of the state hospitals may even increase.

These are some of the salient facts. Where do we go from here?
Shall we ask for the demise of outmoded and "obsolete" hospitals or
shall we look at them as a community resource, needing reshaping? I
believe that the need of mental hospitals as a part of a unified and
purposeful system in the delivery of mental health services is here to
stay.

1. To begin with, not all mental hospitals now in operation are old,
obsolete "psychiatric warehouses" with no links to the surrounding
community. Some have CCMHCs or are part of a federation of associated service facilities comprising nursing home care, sheltered workshops, rehabilitation centers for addicts, treatment centers for children,
etc.

2. A large percentage of the state hospital population is court referred and whether clinicians like it or not, these people must stay in a custodial facility—be it a jail or a mental hospital. Moreover, depending on the legislation in each state, screening of a patient by a community facility to determine whether he can be treated in the community may or may not be possible prior to hospitalization in a state facility. In cases in which no such option for community care prior to hospitalization exists, the hospital is the only resource available for psychiatric offenders.

Finally, there are several groups of mental patients, and certain ones just cannot be released into the community. Among those who can are the patients with what we might call "living problems." These include patients with neuroses, personality disorders, simple schizophrenia, and other diagnoses. A second group includes patients with so-called habit disorders such as alcohol and drug abuse. There is little doubt that most of those in these two groups could be better treated in the community. Indeed, nearly all CCMHCs and ADAMHA-funded drug and alcohol facilities provide treatment facilities for these groups and for others who can benefit from short-term therapy. It is not with these but with the final group that we have problems: This is the group of chronic patients and psychiatric offenders. Their diagnoses include severe schizophrenia, paranoia, severe disease of the senium, some categories of sex offenders, and others who might be harmful to the community and themselves.

Many in this group of chronic patients do not respond even to chemotherapy. That they would do any better in the community is open to question. Psychiatric offenders are judicially referred and must have custodial care anyhow. By taking them out of state hospitals and putting them in jail, the state would be subjecting them to penal rigors and further education in crime, which, although bad enough for the healthy inmates, is even worse for the mentally ill. Even for societal offenders not referred by the courts, such as sex offenders, an argument could be made to keep them in custodial care to protect the community. In my judgment, there will always be a group of persons for whom the state must care, and it is for them that state hospitals are necessary.

Another way of looking at the appropriate utilization of both centralized and community facilities is to examine the overall goals of treatment. Let us start by recognizing that for each decision relating to patients in mental hospitals there are three beneficiaries—the patient, his family, and society as a whole. It is often assumed that the goals of the patient are the goals of the family or society. Yet this is not necessarily so. Take the case of a repeated sex offender. It could be argued that by learning to cope with the strains and pressures in society, he could cure himself. But society's first goal is the protection of its citizens, and society's legal processes may require custodial rather than community care for those seen as dangerous. Even in noncustodial care, the question of benefit to society should be looked into. Suppose it could be proved that a patient would be substantially better in a community setting but with additional costs for treatment. And suppose treatment facilities could be found to deal with his problems. Substantial cost increases for his treatment may reduce the availability of funds for others such as cancer or heart disease victims, etc. In addition, getting someone off "patient" status may save money for the state hospital or Department of Mental Health, but given the unemployability of many patients, they are likely to be transferred to welfare rolls and become wards of the state nonetheless.

If the above logic is accepted—namely, that the hospitals should be a part of an integrated system of mental health delivery services for the catchment area the hospitals are serving—then a systematic approach is required toward the evaluation of community care, development of cost data, etc. I suggest the following specific approaches:

1. A unified treatment plan for patient management of each patient which would involve (a) a tracking system from point of entry to the point of exit in mental health delivery systems; (b) joint responsibility for patient care, even when the patient is released to the community; and (c) a system for exchange of information on the patient's progress.

2. State hospitals, like CCMHCs, should seek multiple funding and establish an accounting system permitting cost–benefit analysis. Most economists will be surprised to learn that cost–benefit analysis is nonexistent in most mental hospitals.

At the state level, what we need is a system study of cost–benefit that would analyze all costs of releasing a patient, such as actual cost reduction in board and treatment; cost of incurred police or legal services; cost to the welfare system; cost to the facility in terms of lost days of work; cost to society in terms of productivity, loss of work days because of critical attack, etc. Similarly, on the benefit side, one must look at the treatment benefit to individuals, the alternative benefit structure for others with equally difficult diseases and in need of funds, the economic benefit to the community through employment of individuals formerly custodially served, the benefit to the facility in terms of availability of a person for family activities, the availability of employment to mental hospitalsworkers, etc.

At the local level, the cost–benefit data need to be analyzed for patients in the state hospitals, for those in nursing homes and boarding houses, for those receiving no care, and for those receiving some care.

In addition, a control group for those receiving the same care in the community as patients receive in the hospital would give reliable cost data.

Thus far, the available cost data does not include such intricate but necessary analyses. A study of 358 released patients from Grafton State Hospital conducted by the Massachusetts Department of Mental Health shows that average nursing home care or boarding house care for those released is $10.15, in contrast to $16.88 per day for the state hospital. However, the figure $10.15 does not include mental health services or medicines for which $1.00 per day was added. While it may be true that the per unit cost of service in the community facility per diem is less than in the state and city hospitals, the longer durations for which persons are cared for in the community settings on a nonchronic diagnosis can result in the cost per episode being substantially higher for the community care overall.

While trying to develop a system to evaluate community care, we should simultaneously develop a new definition of the state hospital. We must get away from the dreary old concept of the state hospital which has been noted for custodial rather than remedial care, for its isolationism, and for its low staff–patient ratio.

A change in the image of state hospitals is already in progress, in fact. Many state hospitals have added outpatient as well as community care services. Many have well-coordinated relationships with CCMHCs. Because of the decline in state hospital populations, the low staff–patient ratios are changing. Young psychiatrists in their first placements are finding work in state hospitals helpful to their careers. Even the isolationism is being dealt with. Many of the state hospitals have halfway houses affiliated with the facility, and many are purchasing facilities in town. The state of South Carolina has adopted a village system in which various apartment buildings can accommodate a limited number of patients.

Furthermore, as suburbia expands, the value of the land on which old state hospitals now stand has gone up ten- to twenty-fold. Most of the buildings, however, are old and dreary and need renovation costing millions, even to bring them up to building code standards. It may be more profitable for the government and the patient to raze such buildings, sell the land, and rent buildings in the community or build new ones. This will help both the continuity-of-care-for-patients concept advocated by many, and the effort to achieve better coordination with legal, judicial, and welfare systems.

Apart from the physical changes, the hospital should be redefined in terms of the goals established for the patients with the advice of the people in the geographic catchment area involved. Joint planning between local programs and state hospitals is necessary. This should employ goal-setting systems for both local facilities and state hospitals. The hospitals should be responsible to locally based policy-making boards and a member of one community's board should serve on the boards of other community-based facilities, and vice versa.

3. Furthermore, one system of funding for local and state programs will help to unify the program. Where state laws do not permit unified funding, a financial contract between a community-based treatment facility and state hospitals should be drawn up, with built-in evaluation to assure the fulfillment of the contract and achievement of treatment goals.

4. Where there is no CCMHC in the area, the state hospital should develop a community system which would involve law enforcement officials, judiciary, clergy, schools, and physicians. This would bring community involvement into the development and evaluation of new services.

There is still no definitive proof as to why community care is better than hospital care. No evaluations of the two systems exist, and it is mostly on faith that I outline here a plan for community care in hospitals. Perhaps state hospital outpatients are different from those CCMHCs served and hence cannot be compared. Perhaps we do not have the methodology to evaluate these two patient groups, or perhaps we do not care to research patient care outcomes? In all research on the closing of state hospitals, little has been done to date on patient care outcome.

In addition, the question that we have answered till now is not where to care for *chronic* patients, but where not to care for them. In order to take care of the chronically disabled, we need a total care system which would see to their housing, use of drugs, training for a job, opportunity to work, and ways to ease the burdens of the community. We are nowhere close to achieving such a total service system.

Of the key considerations outlined above, I believe that the most important concept is evaluation. Objectives, priorities, and ways of measuring progress must be set. We in mental health have never known accountability in terms of demonstrable results. We may have a difficult time achieving such accountability, but in these days of unified health delivery systems, funds will undoubtedly go to the programs which can *demonstrate* results. Some means of evaluation, goal setting, and performance standards, therefore, must be part of the future for all mental health services, including the state hospital.

# Index

Mayhon, J., 58
McKerracher, D. G., 179
McKinley, R. A., 39
Medicaid and Medicare, 151–52, 207, 208
Medical training, hospitals and, 48, 171
Mendel, Werner M., 7, **21–29,** 194, 195
Mendkoff, E., 85, 99
Mendicino State Hospital (Calif.), 4
Mental health center, 11, 206
    quality of care, financing and, 150–51,
        162–63
Mental health movement, 40–41, 134, 143
Michigan, 6
Miller, Dorothy, 118, 163–64
Minnesota, 154–55
Mississippi, 148, 151
Modesto State Hospital, 4, 15, 68, 76, 83–95
Modlin, H. C., 36
Modular programming, 195–96
Morrissey, J., 114
Mortality, posttransfer, 130
    chronically ill, 99–100, 106
    geriatric patients, 89–91, 100
Mosher, L. R., 35

Napa State Hospital, 4, 69
National Institute of Mental Health, 12,
    149
Nelson, R. L., 132
"Neurosis, institutional," 115
*New England Journal of Medicine,* 168
New York City, 36, 134–35, 164
New York State (*see also* New York City),
    18, 36, 38–39, 98–109, 133, 148–49,
    152, 161, 162–63
    Mental Hygiene, Department of, 39, 98
*New York State Association for Retarded
    Children, Inc.* v. *Rockefeller,* 148–49
*New York Times,* 164
North Carolina, 154
Number of closings, 9–10
Nursing homes, 88, 89, 208

*Oakes* case, 153
Oberleder, M., 134–35
Ohio, 5, 206
Osmond, Humphrey, 180

Partlow State School and Hospital, 168
Pasamanick, B., 195
Pasamanick, E., 54

Patient sitters, 22
Patients, impact of closings on, 75, 79,
    83–109, 128–30
    chronically ill, 72–73, 98–108
    elderly, 18, 83–95
    transfer trauma, reducing, 130–32
    *see also* Relocation of patients; specific
        facilities and services
Peer groups, 22
Pennsylvania, 6, 36–37, 154
Performance standards, 212
Perlmutter, F., 51
Pinel, 115
Plant and buildings, 211
Plog, Stanley C., **3–8**
Political aspects of closings, 17, 66–68,
    119–23
    autonomy, professional, and, 137–38
Pollack, E. S., 49
Population, hospitals, 14–15, 45–46, 54,
    98, 128, 168, 178–79, 206
    cost/patient ratios, 78–79
    diagnostic distribution of admissions,
        207–8
    discharge, criteria and rate of, 100–4
    reduction of, Saskatchewan program
        and, 179–90
    staff ratios, 168–70, 206, 211
Problems and conditions in state
    hospitals, 6, 16–17, 165–66
    Comprehensive Community Mental
        Health Centers compared, 50–55
    environment, negative aspects of, 21–
        27, 115–17
    psychiatry, judicial intervention and,
        166–73
Professional staff and employees, 5, 48
    hospital reform, judicial intervention
        and, 166–73
    impact of closings, 4, 68–70, 74–78
    opposition to closings, 4–5, 17, 18, 79,
        128–29, 194–95
    patient ratios, 168–70, 206, 211
    patients and reactions of, 75
    right to help, usurpation of, 57–58
    shortage of, 108–69
    understanding of closure, 70, 74–75,
        79–80
*Psychiatric Annals,* 160
*Psychiatric News,* 19, 168
*Psychiatric Viewpoint,* 157